THE SOBER Leap

Table of Contents

"The sun calls us out of the shadows
to leap into the light and feel it's warm embrace.
Inviting us to find ourselves again."
—The Author

Prologue

In the throes of addiction, you broke promises on a daily basis. You committed to stop more times than not, only to find yourself staring in the mirror the morning after, with one more reason to doubt it would ever be possible to live any other way.

Until the day you were forced to take action. You fell to your knees and finally surrendered. You tossed your feet into the fire and held them there. You squirmed and moaned as you watched the flames burn your toes. Pounding your fists and raising holy hell, you waited for the ashes to cool.

As the pain subsided, life peeked over the horizon to greet you. Challenging you to face your demons and little by little, to

let them go. Offering you a shift in perspective and a chance to create a different story.

Now your arms are open wide and you're ready to take it all in. To release the fear and self-doubt that's been holding you back. To discover your inner strength and reawaken to the beauty surrounding you.

You're poised to step into a bigger, bolder life, full of love and unwavering self-acceptance. Reaching beyond who you are today and embracing who you are meant to become.

The time has come to raise the stakes and make a personal commitment of grand proportions.

To leap out of the shadows and into your own magnificence.

Introduction

Admitting I was addicted to alcohol was as unanticipated as a sudden grope from a creepy guy on a crowded dance floor. By the time I realized what was actually happening, his sweaty hand was on my ass and a slimy, wet kiss had landed smack on my lips. Leaving me spinning in a mix of disgust, embarrassment, and total confusion.

It took all the strength I had to take that first step. To stare down the truth after years of denial, and finally admit I had a problem. I was living a comfortable life, had a successful career, and by all accounts, could have gone on drinking myself to death without anyone even noticing. My secret struggles with

alcohol were kept hidden for two reasons. I was a good liar and I drank alone.

After spending over a decade drinking myself into a dark and passive haze, trying to temper the noise in my life, I woke up one morning with a deafening pain between my ears and a faint voice telling me it was finally time to stop the crazy. That was my moment.

By the time I finally quit, there had been no one telling me it was time to stop. So, when I finally did, the validation from friends and family that I longed for was virtually non-existent. Those I confided in about my struggle tried their best to empathize, but for the most part had no idea things had gotten so out of hand. They'd never seen me falling down at a party or missing days of work. I was discreet with my pain and waited until I was home, alone, and out of view to come undone.

I think they remained more perplexed than relieved about my decision to stop simply because they didn't see it. I've had to make peace with that and rather than let it discourage me, I've found that it only strengthens my resolve to seek out support from those who understand my struggle and commitment to my recovery.

Looking back, my first six months of sobriety were a total blur. I can remember counting the days, with one goal in mind, to get past 6pm without a drink. That was considered success. I

knew only one thing to be true. Time was my healer and it was all I had to count on to keep me going.

As the days went on, I began to feel better physically, but underneath I was lost in the same old thought patterns I'd been holding onto since well before my life spun out of control. The booze was gone, but the pain and doubt had a hold on me and were refusing to let go.

I needed support, but didn't look to the rooms of AA to find it. I'd attended a few meetings early on, but I never felt at home there. So, I decided to seek out community in smaller recovery groups and forums. To my surprise, among the many amazing people I met, there were a significant number of women who admitted they felt the same way—disoriented, stuck, and unable to figure out how to make things better.

Here we were, on the other side of our battle with addiction, trying to live up to the expectations of everyone around us, and somehow we felt gypped. Where was the bliss of recovery we'd heard so much about? Were we missing something? We found ourselves back on the same roller coaster ride of trying to be the best loving partners, caregivers, career women, and impeccable multitaskers we could be, feeling virtually paralyzed by relentless thoughts of the past, fears of the future and an inability to find joy in our present.

Now don't get me wrong, as you know it's amazing to be free from the clutches of addiction, but when you pop out the

other end, the world you return to doesn't exactly welcome you with open arms. Even for those of us who have incredible friends and family, they are not typically set up to support us upon re-entry. It's like a new set of rules have been established overnight and no one received the playbook.

So, we're left to our own devices to assimilate as best we can back into the same circle of chaos we left. Only this time we're facing even more challenging terrain. It's like trekking the Himalayas with no provisions. Not exactly a set up for survival.

Once sober, we're often caught in the dilemma of putting ourselves first in order to heal, while facing the fear and anxiety of falling back into old habits as we struggle to meet the same set of expectations that fueled our addiction in the first place. The stress of coping under the pressures of career, family, and relationships only increases the challenge. The anesthesia is gone and here we are, naked and confused, without a clue of how to deal with this new and raw way of living.

To add to the mix, there are additional pressures placed on us every day that add to the complexity. To name a few:

Tipsy World

I like to start with this one because I think it's the most pervasive. From the moment we step foot into recovery we're faced with the challenge of being consistently exposed to the substance that brought us down. It's all around us and if we are not careful, can trigger us, especially when we are feeling particularly vulnerable. Unless we're living in a highly controlled environment, this requires us to remain steadfast and diligent in our commitment to our sobriety at all times to prevent temptation or potential relapse.

Social Life

Getting back into the social scene can be a huge challenge. The first thing that came to my mind when I first got sober was *I will never go out again.* Extreme, I know, but having laid awake several nights in college in a full on panic when my fake ID was stolen, thinking fun as I knew it had come to a screeching halt, this was a very big deal. The energy it takes to even fathom, let alone take the necessary steps to rebuild a life without alcohol feels daunting, especially in the early stages, when trying to simply get through the day can be a struggle.

Circles of Influence

Although we may not want to admit it, in recovery we find that our current circle of non-sober friends most likely won't have a clue about what we're experiencing. Particularly if they are the ones who drank with us in the first place. This could be a partner, spouse, family member, or friend who may want you back in the game with them, not out at some café having a deep conversation with some yoga dude over a cup of Chamomile tea. Their visual, not ours. They miss us, and their intentions may be good, but they can end up inadvertently sabotaging our recovery if we're not careful.

Communication

Like it or not, there's a stigma around addiction and "coming out" to the world in sobriety can require an exhausting amount of messaging to others regarding who we are now versus who we used to be. Unless we just choose to ignore it, we may find ourselves directly, or indirectly, justifying our choice to be sober on a fairly regular basis. This takes an enormous amount of time, mental energy, and patience on our part, especially during the difficult days.

The unspoken truth is that no one has the perfect answer for how to "do" recovery. We stop drinking, do our best to find support, and avoid getting triggered. There are few rules to follow with the exception of one—to stay sober. The steps to this sassy little rumba called sobriety can be a challenge, especially for those of us who are looking for a more holistic plan for sustained recovery.

Back to the Basics

As we begin to recognize these obstacles, it's difficult to feel like the odds are stacked in our favor and things can get pretty discouraging. It's no wonder we feel disoriented as we get thrown back into this spin cycle of life. Things can go sideways quickly unless we have a solid foundation to steady our footing.

As I took a closer look at this dilemma, a question came to mind. Could it be that the guidance we are all so desperately looking for is right in front of our eyes? Maybe our success is not achieved by changing the situation around us, but by doing the internal work necessary to reach a new level of awareness about ourselves and our own capabilities. This would require us to peel away the excess layers of self-doubt that we've been hiding behind and re-activate our own inner compass to find the answers.

These layers run deep and are accumulated over time, so it would involve getting back to the basics and wiggling loose the habits and behaviors that we've learned over the years. In doing this, it could unlock so many of the challenges we face, by creating space for our inner wisdom to come through and letting it take the lead—transporting us from a place of restriction to one of expansion. Untethered by any preconceived notion we had in the past about who we are or who others think we're supposed to be.

With these basics in mind, the Leap Truths were born. A simple set of guiding principles that invite you to fundamentally shift how you operate, stripping away the doubt and empowering you to show up with unapologetic strength and confidence. Focusing on areas that can be particularly challenging to practice even without addiction at play, you'll find that once you develop these new behaviors, you'll begin to see a significant change in all aspects of your life.

The 11 Truths are:

- Surrender
- Feel the Force
- Dig Deep
- Stay Present
- Crush the Bubble
- Sing Mama Sing!
- Breathe
- Take Care
- Moxie Baby
- Find the Spark
- Bring it

As we delve into these in greater detail in the following chapters, you'll learn about the energy that surrounds and protects you, and the importance of finding your voice to speak up and be heard. We'll dig into the power of choice and letting go of past behaviors to embrace the here and now. I'll introduce you to a proven model that strengthens the connection between your thoughts, feelings, and the circumstances you create in your life. We'll also discuss how to nourish your body and use movement to overcome emotional blocks, and explore ways to cultivate your own creativity and discover your purpose, so you can share your experiences and gifts with the world.

Lastly, we'll identify the typical roadblocks you may encounter that steer you away from showing up fully, and provide you with the tools to overcome them.

At the end of each chapter, I'll be highlighting what blocks us, thoughts you may consider adopting to support new habits and practices you can start incorporating on a daily basis.

It's important to note, that these concepts are nothing new. In fact, they're merely a collection of basic truths you've known all along, but by either social conditioning or learned experience, have lost along the way. My hope is to bring them into crystal clear focus so they become second nature, and the primary foundation for you to thrive in your sobriety.

Before we get started on our journey together, I'd like to acknowledge the remarkable courage and strength of character you've demonstrated by exploring new ways to enhance your experience in recovery. Having picked up this book, you've already made a significant leap forward in creating positive change.

Although you may have seen your addiction as a burden in the past, it's now time to turn your experience into something not only positive, but life affirming and the impetus for powerful transformation.

I only ask one thing. That you remain open to the ideas presented in the book and promise me that you will take what works for you and leave the rest.

That's the beautiful thing about life after all, we always have choice.

Chapter One

Surrender

It will set you free.

I suck at telling the truth, I thought to myself as I found my way to the corner table and waited for my sister to arrive. Mary and I decided to meet at her favorite Mediterranean restaurant on College Ave. I told her that dinner was "my treat," knowing this was just my way of adding levity to an otherwise grueling situation. It was my only way to distract myself from the fact that I was getting ready to serve my heart and soul to her on a platter of Spanakopita, and although I loved her and knew she loved me, my fear of rejection was weighing on me like nothing I'd ever felt before.

I sat down at the table, staring at the door as people continued to file in. I reached down to grab my phone in an attempt to keep myself busy and could feel the cool of my sweaty palms sticking to the case. After what seemed like an eternity, I finally saw her walk in and make her way across the room.

She gave me a tight hug and reached back to pull off her jacket. This was rare for her to leave my niece with her stepdaughter on a weeknight. Thinking this was just another one of our evenings out to catch up, she was a bit giddy. I tried to match her energy but struggled to keep up the front.

We glanced over the menu and as I stared at the page, I found myself repeating in my head *tell the truth, tell the truth* as if the repetition of those simple words would automatically make it happen. But I knew better. In many ways the truth and I had barely met and falling in step with this distant acquaintance of mine was already feeling awkward.

As we caught up on my niece, her new school, and what her step kids were up to, a lull came in the conversation and she blurted out "so what's been going on with you?"

This was it. The defining moment where I spill my guts and watch my life as a normal person pass before my very eyes. Like a freight train, it was coming toward me and the pit in my stomach gave way to a loud ringing in my ears. I was paralyzed as my heart grew heavy and I could feel the heat of the blood rushing to my face.

I didn't know where to look and I knew if we made eye contact, I would lose my courage altogether, so I focused my eyes on a painting on the wall directly behind her and suddenly blurted out "I actually have something I wanted to talk to you about." She sat back calmly with no anticipation of anything unusual and said "Oh, yeah? What's up?"

My pulse was racing now as I forced myself to stay in the moment and fumbled to find the words. As if on cue, the laughter from the table next to us raised in pitch right as I blurted out "I've decided to stop drinking." Instantly, I felt my stomach tighten. *How could I be so stupid!* Mustering up the courage to say the words "I'm an alcoholic" was so far out of reach that when it came to my moment of truth, I knew I blew it. It felt surreal. I was sitting outside of my body watching the conversation unfold.

My twisted logic told me that if I couched it as a simple decision to change a bothersome little habit like say, cutting out salt or giving up gluten, the magnitude of what was happening would somehow dissolve in the moment. But the words just lay there on the table, waiting for her to respond.

My sister and I grew up in a family where drinking was a part of our everyday life.

My father was a drinker, but never felt the need to explain it or label it. It just was what it was. Being Irish Catholic, alcohol has been tightly woven into the fabric of our family for generations. I learned early on that drinking was the best way to cope with the ups and downs of life. Regardless of how destructive it may become.

Although it caused a great deal of angst for me growing up, ironically, as I grew older, it became the first thing I reached for to provide me with a sense of comfort and ease. Needless to say, my relationship with alcohol has been complicated from the start.

As I found myself at this strange intersection between denial and acceptance, I was far more comfortable putting off the truth when it came to my own demons. So as this moment fell upon me, I felt my fear of disclosure tenfold. It was as if somehow confessing that I had a problem, was indirectly calling attention to an extended family dynamic that was better left alone.

My sister had been in recovery for over 20 years and had kept her sobriety fairly quiet around our family. She didn't share too much about it and although we all showed our love and support, we made a point not to ask too many questions. An Irish skill we'd honed was keeping things light and breezy regardless of what was beneath the surface. I knew deep down for years that I was fighting the same battle as she was, but never had the courage to usher in the conversation.

I started to explain how I'd been hiding my drinking for years, that I drank alone every night, and that I felt like I was dying inside. I expected her to say *I was wondering when you were finally going to stop.* Instead she looked me straight in the eye and said, *I seriously had no idea.* Suddenly things came to an abrupt halt in my mind and I knew she was in total shock. The truth was finally out. I was officially stepping out of the shadows and into the light with her.

I told her I was scared and confused and that I had no clue how to do this. She smiled and looked me square in the eye and said something that has stuck with me to this day.

Don't you realize? This is when the good stuff starts.

From that day forward, I've come to understand exactly what she meant and know beyond the shadow of a doubt that in order to release what life had in store for me, I had to let go of my secrets and start telling the truth.

Truth

Ironically, truth is the first thing to greet us in recovery. Which is pretty remarkable. It's been waiting for us to show up for years and although we've spent much of our lives skirting and hiding behind it, it still gives us a big bear hug when we walk in the door. It knows in its heart of hearts that it's finally time for us to make amends.

In the beginning, truth takes us a while to even recognize. Especially when we haven't been around it for a long time, but it's so integral to the success of our recovery that there's no getting around it. You can try to fight it but in the end if you're serious about your recovery, you'll need to surrender to it once and for all.

I felt a sense of freedom when I finally let truth back into my life. It started the day I got sober and I literally felt the monkey climb off my back. When people ask what I'm most grateful for when it comes to my recovery, I say the joy of waking up without a hangover (that is definitely #1!), and finally letting go of all the lies.

The first step is holding ourselves responsible for our own actions and decisions. This may feel strange at first since we are out of practice, but it's necessary as we come into our own as sober individuals. Living a lie can be incredibly exhausting and if we're going to operate at a higher frequency, which we will delve into further in the next chapter, we need to be relentlessly open, honest, and accountable.

The BS

The truth is too difficult for me. If I tell the truth, I'm only going to disappoint others and lower their expectations of me. I have a difficult time letting other people in, so it's just easier to tell a white lie. I'm a very private person, so I don't feel compelled to let others in on my secrets.

Blockers

We can always come up with a good reason to withhold the truth in life. The expectations of others or commitments we make may feel like they are forcing us to decide between telling a white lie or potentially letting others down. Sometimes the latter feels unbearable and causes us to compromise. We may also have grown up with many secrets, so it has become a way of life to keep others at a safe distance.

The Shift

I need to make the conscious choice to tell the truth. It is my own integrity at stake. Once I can stand strong in who I am and all of the complexities that go with it, I will open myself up to so much more in life. Meeting others from a place of truth encourages them to do the same and only deepens my relationship with myself and others.

Daily Practice

Write down the secrets you're keeping and the consequences of revealing them. As you examine what comes up, you begin to realize that it's a story you're telling yourself and it's yours to be re-written.

Then write down the little white lies you may have told yourself or others during the course of a day or week. Why did you feel the urge to do so? Once you start to deconstruct each of them, you begin to see that this learned behavior is merely a habit, and once interrupted with closer examination can be changed.

If being a person of integrity is important to you, regardless of how visible it is to others, telling the truth is the only way to achieve it.

Chapter Two

Feel the Force
It's all around you.

Lake Michigan, 1982

I felt the crack split slowly beneath my feet as it gave way and I plunged into the dark freezing water. *Grab my camera!* I shouted as the weight of my wool coat got heavy and my body sunk deeper into the lake.

I looked up at my friend standing just a few feet above me and threw my bag onto the solid block of ice, reaching up to grab hold of her sleeve. I could feel my legs start to tingle and the whipping wind sting my face. It was dark and the only light

I could see was a slight shimmer reflecting off of the surface of the water.

As I started to panic, I tried to will myself weightless. She clenched my arm and after two failed attempts, hoisted me up with her full body weight, pulling me onto the ice beside her. We lay on our backs looking up at the sky, shivering and out of breath. Running back to the car, she scrambled to turn on the heat as we sank into the front seat. I turned to her and with a sigh, mouthed *what the f***?* She glanced back at me with a look of terror and a nervous laugh. We drove home in silence.

She dropped me off and I ran upstairs to my bedroom as fast as I could to take off my soaking wet clothes and hide the evidence. Knowing in my heart, I could never breathe a word.

I contemplated telling my mom, but knew right away it was a bad idea. Knowing she would react in utter dismay *Oh, for crying out loud Noelle, what were you two doing out there in the first place?* Her aggravation at my carelessness would surely overshadow any sense of relief she may have had that I was ok. It was confirmed, I couldn't tell a soul.

I lay awake that night staring up at the ceiling, feeling scared, confused, and completely alone. The shock was wearing off and the enormity of what had happened had started to sink in. Running through the chain of events in my head, trying to make sense of it all, I kept telling myself, *we'd only been out there for twenty minutes or so. Just getting a few shots in for my class before the sun went down. What's the big deal?*

I bet I was under water for no more than 90 seconds, but the memory of that experience has haunted me for over 30 years. Wondering why the universe had allowed me to be so reckless, dangling me over the edge of death like that, only to snap me back in an instant to carry on like nothing had ever happened.

I knew in my heart that there was something undeniable that spared me that night beneath the icy cold water of Lake Michigan. It was shaking me to wake up and recognize the fragility of my life and although I had no clue how to make sense of it at the time, it was my first glimpse of a force outside of myself, lifting me up and out of danger. It was powerful and protective, and although I had no idea what it was, I was overwhelmingly grateful for its presence.

The next time I would feel that force was on November 25, 2011. The day I got sober. I sat on the corner of my bed, feeling beyond exhausted, wondering how things had gotten so bad. My life had gone from manageable to completely out of control in what felt like a hot minute and this time, there was no one to save me but myself. I was at the end of my rope. This was it. This secret, amongst the thousands that I had accumulated in my life up to that point, was one that I could no longer keep.

For the previous eight years, I had woken up every morning with a crushing hangover. In sickness and in health, I never missed a day of work or a day of drinking. My relationship with alcohol was steadfast and true. I would stumble to the bathroom and as I stared in the mirror, looking at the pain in my eyes, I'd hear a faint voice telling me I was beyond help and destined to remain stuck in a life of shame and addiction. I was lost and thought I had no way out.

For some reason, that day turned out to be different from the others. I could feel a vibration in my body and the voice was telling me that if I didn't stop, I was going to die. Through the fog of my weary brain, without a doubt I knew this to be true.

From that day forward, the presence I felt in that moment has never left me. It has taken up residence in my soul and I feel its support and protection as I continue to gain the wisdom to make better choices in my life. Its power is undeniable and I know it will always be with me. I am never alone.

Force Field

The universe provides us all with a force that guides us through the peaks and valleys of our lives. Call it what you want but it's an energy that surrounds us. It's our own personal steward that keeps us safe and in step with life, but it takes will on our part to help it guide us and lead us in the right direction. This force has been present since the day we were born. It just takes some of us more time to wake up and recognize it.

For most of us in recovery, this is especially true. Our senses have become so dulled by addiction that we're unable to tap into this energy consistently until we awaken within ourselves in sobriety. As we get more quiet and in tune with our surroundings, we become more aware of its presence in our midst. This also allows us to see our past with different eyes and recognize its hand in those experiences, so we can no longer ignore its existence.

Source Energy

This powerful force is fueled by energy. Energy can't be seen but it's all around us. It's inherently vibrational, and everything in existence has a high or low vibration. Your energetic vibration is controlled by your emotions. When you have emotions that feel good, you are vibrating at a high level. This is when you're aligned with your Source Energy.

When you experience emotions that make you feel stuck, anxious, fearful etc., you are vibrating at a low level or outside the natural flow of Source. Being out of flow, as you are more frequently in addiction, makes it increasingly more difficult to connect with this vital force around you.

That's why it's so critical in recovery to let go of anxiety, anger, and negativity so we can regain balance and call in these powerful forces. Our goal is to vibrate at a high frequency on a consistent basis because what we focus on expands. Once we make the choice to rise above the fray and accept the invitation to change our mindset and let go, the universe starts to dance with us.

By raising and aligning our vibration with that of Source, or being in flow, we are connecting with that power that is among us and can restore our balance and well-being. We know we're in alignment when things come together effortlessly and we feel a momentum and pull toward living life authentically.

Along with checking your negativity at the door, it's vital to remain in a constant state of gratitude. This may feel like a tall order to some of you, if you feel you've been dealt a s*** hand, but it's time to turn that thinking around. The experiences you've had are what made you the incredible woman you are today, with depth and understanding that you wouldn't have if you hadn't gone through the experience of addiction. Realizing the order of things is just the beginning, and saying thank you for all that you have and all that you want to bring into your life is laying the groundwork for incredible change. We'll be addressing our ability to release negativity in Chapter 5 when we dig further into thought work.

Signs

Once you start to gain alignment, you will begin noticing little things that come into your presence that tell you, you are in flow. It may sound far-fetched, but you will have experiences show up in your life that are just what you need at just the right time. Pay attention to them. They are not merely coincidence. They are signs that indicate you are in balance with this life affirming element. When you make this connection with Source and recognize the guidance of an energy outside of yourself, you become virtually unstoppable.

So how do you release the power of these forces in your life? It's easy. Increase your vibration by reframing your thoughts and letting go of the need to control the outcomes in your life. Once you let the universe do its thing, the magic will happen.

Much like in our drinking days, when we tried to control everything around us, we like to think that we are the only ones who have a hand in what's at play in this life. We soon realize that there is so much more out there conspiring to make things happen. There is nothing more powerful than the belief that the universe will provide and wants the best for us. Once we shift our focus on letting go and letting things happen without meddling, that's when our life will start to light up.

To align yourself with a greater power, in whatever form that takes for you, means to simply surrender to the uncertainty and have faith in the power of this force that is here to guide you and pave the way for you to contribute at a much higher level in the world.

All you need to do is let it.

The BS

I'm alone in all of this. I have no support and the universe has put this crap in front of me to teach me a lesson. I'm not worthy of happiness. If I was, I wouldn't have had this addiction in the first place. I control my life and there are no outside forces doing anything for me.

Blockers

There may be people in your life who don't believe in internal or external forces having anything to do with the outcomes in your life and that is perfectly OK. In fact, you may be thinking that way yourself. In the past, you've undoubtedly experienced challenges that could make you disbelieve there is a universe that pulls for you to succeed, but I ask you to reserve judgment and just start noticing. After all, you've stopped a deadly addiction that has taken down millions of others from claiming your own life. Was that just dumb luck? I don't think so.

The Shift

The universe is here to serve. Even in my darkest days, it was putting in front of me the circumstances that have led me here today. I am wiser because of it. The key to success is accepting that I have the power to create my own experience and it's NOT about doing.

The universe is loving and supportive, safe and generous. It will be there to guide me on this journey. All I need to do is step out of the way and let it all unfold.

Daily Practice

Start paying closer attention to daily signs of support and love from the universe. It can be as simple as a comment made by a friend or a situation falling into place in all the right ways, letting you know that you made the right decision.

The best way to tap into the force around you is to let go of judgment and expectation about how your life needs to be. Once you decide to stop pushing against life to try to control every outcome, the game will change completely.

Start keeping a journal and write at least one paragraph a night before going to bed. Take note of how your day unfolded. Highlight the things that went well and those that didn't. Were there any coincidences or incidents that were noteworthy? I guarantee, as you become more conscious of it, you will start to see synchronicities you never saw before and begin to understand how the greater force in our lives truly guides us in the choices each and every day.

Say "thank you". Every day. Not only for the blessings you already have in your life but for those you want to create. Acting as if you already have them will keep you in a place of abundance and open you up to receiving so much more.

Chapter Three

Dig Deep

Honor your feelings. They're your best teachers.

I wish I could say my moment of clarity came in a flash,
but it didn't. It was a gradual process that involved a failed
attempt to get sober in 2005 right before my niece was
born. I was determined to put my addiction aside and be fully
present and a positive role model for this new little bundle we
were welcoming into our family. Along came Gracie and two
years of blissful sobriety.

Then I met Mark. I know now that I was still in deep denial
and naively hoped that a new relationship might change things

for the better. I was good at avoiding the topic of sobriety at all costs, so I justified my relapse as an inevitability since no one had really noticed I'd stopped in the first place. I just thought *screw it* and hopped back on the hamster wheel.

Mark was picture perfect at first. Well sort of. He was funny and engaging and seemed to have his act together, until he'd had a few drinks, at which point he'd become a complete asshole. It turned out, he had a more voracious penchant for drinking than I did, along with a whole host of abandonment and anger issues that began to slowly reveal themselves shortly after we started dating.

It was a winning combination for a girl like me, who was more than ready to jump back into my own little form of dating torture and try to work my magic on yet another self-loathing charmer who couldn't find his way out of a paper bag, let alone participate in a relationship.

Switching into "fix it" mode was my forte and a great way to avoid the real time and attention I should have been giving myself. As one would predict, the drama brought my drinking to the forefront and I was back in the circus for one more round of crazy with my brand new shiny boyfriend.

The interesting thing about my relationship with Mark was that his erratic behavior got so close to absurd that at times, I could actually feel myself floating above the situation looking at it as an observer. I was so out to lunch emotionally, that if you asked me how I felt about him at any given time, I would have honestly struggled to find an answer. I was literally just a passenger on an old dilapidated bus, heading down a dark bumpy road, along for the ride.

Needless to say, I was oblivious to the signs. I can recall one Friday evening instead of picking me up, he asked me to meet him out at a bar *(red flag #1)* and much to my dismay, he had been drinking since about 3pm *(red flag #2)*. Mark was in sales and worked from home, which not only allowed him to complain endlessly about his boss not appreciating him, but it gave him license to cut out mid-day for a 4 hour lunch and call it "working" *(red flag #3)*.

I could tell when I got there, by his sharp responses and inability to master the English language, that he had been well over served and was getting increasingly more agitated. I'd found after some time, that he would get melancholy on beer and nasty on the hard stuff (red flag #4). Regardless of where we were going, the destination was always a booze-drenched monologue about how nobody respected him. *(OK, enough with the red flags already, you get the idea!)*

After downing a few drinks of my own, I decided that the only way to salvage the evening was to get some food in him to lift his mood, so we walked down the block to a Japanese restaurant. After ordering, I tried to make the conversation light and mentioned that I was going to start training for a marathon.

Instead of the expected response of "oh, how cool, what a great challenge" or "that's wonderful, I'll come watch," he looked at me as if he was going to throw a punch across the table and as plain as day he snapped.

He began yelling "Oh, REALLY?! Well, I don't know about you, but I actually WANT to be in a relationship!!" I would try to interject and he began talking over me as the two tables next to us stared in disbelief. "Fine, go ahead and spend your time training, run your f*** marathon!" At that point, I began to get up from the table, praying he would stop. My mind went blank and I actually didn't hear anything after that other than my own voice saying "This just got creepy, I need to leave."

As I made my way down the block to my car, he began running after me shouting "You think I'M creepy? I think YOU'RE creepy!" The whole scene felt surreal. As if I'd been asleep at the wheel and suddenly woke up to being chased down the street by a raging lunatic. This could not be someone I actually chose to date. Had I been even remotely conscious of what was going on with myself internally, I would have stated my needs in the moment and set a boundary. In hindsight, if I'd had a clue how to do this, I would have done so much earlier in the relationship and could have avoided the sidewalk drama all together, but suffice it to say, in the moment, I was paralyzed.

True to form, on my drive home, I made an attempt to tease out any strand of co-dependent logic I could get my hands on. *Is the marathon threatening him? Is it the time I would spend training that got him so upset?* I was always so good at blaming myself, but this time I couldn't do it. I realized that in the fog, I had unknowingly walked into this strange and aggressive territory and had no idea how to find my way out of it.

I was so stunned that I stopped my car and whispered to myself *how the hell did I get here?* I knew right then and there, that I needed to stop being passive and start participating in my life. It would not be until I stopped drinking for the final time that following year, that I could fully embrace it and take action.

I learned so much from the relationships I found myself in during my drinking days. Looking back on them, I realize that I not only didn't allow myself access to my feelings, but I actively rejected them and pushed them away. Leaving no room for even the most well intended of partners to enter this inner sanctum of obliviousness I had created.

A critical step in maintaining a healthy sober life is accessing our feelings and expressing the needs that come up as a result. This isn't easy for a majority of us who have spent our lives denying our feelings in an effort to make them go away. The reality is, in order to remain free from addiction, we need to pay attention to our emotions on a daily basis so we don't fall back on our old habit of finding external vices to mask them.

Acknowledging our internal cues gives us access to what feels right or wrong at any given time. We need to let go of the fear that these feelings may somehow overwhelm us if we bring them to the surface. This couldn't be farther from the truth. The more familiar we become with our feelings, the more we realize that they provide us with so much vital information. They are our teachers and the gateway that opens us up to connecting to ourselves and others on a much deeper level.

Checking Out

When I was in high school, I wrote my junior theme on a brilliant and extremely hopeful book by Viktor Frankl, *Man's Search For Meaning*. It was life changing. Frankl was a Holocaust survivor who spent time as an inmate in the Auschwitz concentration camp.

After surviving this horrific experience, he conducted an analysis on how human beings cope with traumatic circumstances. He found that after going through the initial phases of shock and apathy, once liberated, many of the inmates experienced a psychological state known as de-personalization. This is a lack of self-awareness that can bring about dissociation from the mind or body.

In early recovery we can find ourselves in a similar state. We've given up the substance, but we continue to look for opportunities to numb out in order to cope. It leaves us feeling disjointed and unable to access our feelings, emotional state, and at times our physical needs.

As we know, our addictive behavior allowed us to check out for years or even decades, and for a good majority of us this happened during our younger years which was a time when our brain functioning was still developing.

So, it's no surprise that when we find ourselves entering recovery, we are a bit disheveled and out of sorts. It's like coming out of the movies in broad daylight. Having been ensconced in the darkness of the theatre, the door suddenly opens and we're out on the street in the bright sunlight. It takes time for our eyes to adjust.

Accessing Feelings

Recognizing and honoring how we feel is a direct result of paying attention to our basic wants and needs. When we decide to ignore them, we are violating ourselves on the deepest level. We are saying to ourselves that our internal balance and comfort are to be ignored and we don't matter.

Accessing feelings can be tricky, especially if we don't have much practice. For those of us who spent most of our life pushing them away, it can feel completely foreign to look inside to identify what is coming up at any given moment.

The first step in accessing our feelings is the willingness to do so. In my own experience, it took a crazy confrontation to shake me into finally owning how I felt and accepting that I needed to start paying attention and participating in my life.

For those of us whose feelings have been disregarded or weren't given permission to show their feelings as a child, this may be a new muscle we need to flex.

Speaking of which, strangely enough it starts with our body. The best way to access your feelings is in recognizing the physical sensation associated with it. When you feel embarrassed or angry, your face may seem hot or turn red. When you are scared or anxious, you may get a sinking feeling—in the pit of your stomach. When you feel happy, you might get a flutter in your chest or a chill down our back.

There may be times when you don't immediately know how you're feeling. It takes practice to consistently recognize what's coming up for you in any given moment. Once you make the connection physically, you can go deeper into what you need in order to respond to it.

Breath work is critical in this process because it calms your senses so you can pay closer attention to what is happening in your body, especially at times when you need to make a request in response to the feeling. We will practice more around the magic of breath work in Chapter 7.

Movement is also helpful in stirring emotion up and out. We don't want feelings to fester because they will make their home in our bodies. The energy from our feelings can lodge in our muscles and organs causing a whole host of issues for us. This can show up even years after the fact. Have you ever heard the expression "your issues are in your tissues?" You may have experienced a yoga class where you feel blocked or stuck in certain poses. This is your body holding onto emotion.

Once we recognize particular feelings and how they manifest, we become less fearful of them surfacing. The good news is that feelings like anger or anxiety typically pass within several minutes, so the key is to learn to acknowledge them and let them run their course.

Bringing feelings up and out is the key to creating a more positive relationship with your internal state regardless of the outside circumstances and more effectively managing your own emotional health.

The BS

I've never been one to share my feelings. I don't really have anything to give. I feel numb and I'm not sure I want to connect with others, in the past it's brought me pain. I often think it's better to just keep my distance and stay on the surface, it's much safer that way.

Blockers

If you've had a history of ignoring your feelings or were conditioned to do so when you were younger, it's a challenge at first to get used to connecting with your feelings and expressing them. Just know that it will take time and practice to create a new way of approaching how you handle them when they come up.

In doing so, others may not be as receptive to listening to what you have to say. Typically, if someone is used to you behaving a certain way, your openness and candor may come as a surprise. Rest assured that this is human nature and changing the paradigm can feel awkward at first. Continuing down this path will increase your confidence and bring forth those around you who understand and fully support your growth in this area.

The Shift

Expressing myself is part of the human experience. It's what I am here to do. My past may have led me down a path of avoidance, but it's time to reclaim my inner truth and let it be known. It's a critical component to forming healthy bonds and relationships and opens me up to receive the love and acceptance I deserve.

Daily Practice

What really helped me as I started this inward journey was meditation. I know you may want to cringe when I say this, because meditation can be challenging for some of us, but it is one of the best ways to quiet the mind and become more aware of your body. It's the key to finding your breath and the best way to begin to recognize those subtleties in our bodies that may be otherwise overlooked when the external world gets too noisy.

This may sound counterintuitive because we have always been told that meditation is a means to calm the body and in deep practice, you are encouraged to refrain from distraction by any sensations that may come up.

This still holds true, but in the stillness, we are training ourselves to become the observer and that is exactly what we want to do with our feelings. Observe without judgment and notice the associated sensations in the body when they appear.

Find time in the mornings or evenings before you go to bed to sit in stillness. Start with 2 minutes and build up your tolerance. It will do wonders for your self-awareness.

Another practice is in the moment when an emotion arises. The best way to start is in a state that is comfortable, either by yourself or with a friend. As soon as you feel a trigger and the sensation begins, write down a description of the physical sensations you are having. If any of you are familiar with a body scan, it is a similar concept. Name the feeling. Does your head ache? Does your forehead seem warm? Does your throat feel heavy? Once you have described this, look at the "feelings sheet" on the next page and identify what best describes how you are feeling in that moment.

At this point, write down what it is you need in order to respond to this feeling. Do you need a few minutes to yourself to step away from the situation? Do you need to make a request of someone else? This may seem difficult at first, but the more you practice, the better you get at accessing, identifying and asking for what you need.

FEELINGS LIST

AMAZED	ANGRY	ANNOYED
ANXIOUS	ASHAMED	BITTER
BORED	COMFORTABLE	CONFUSED
CONTENT	DEPRESSED	DETERMINED
DISDAIN	DISGUSTED	EAGER
EMBARRASSED	ENERGETIC	ENVIOUS
EXCITED	FOOLISH	FRUSTRATED
FURIOUS	GRIEVING	HAPPY
HOPEFUL	HURT	INADEQUATE
INSECURE	INSPIRED	IRRITATED
JEALOUS	JOYFUL	LONELY
LOST	LOVING	MISERABLE
MOTIVATED	NERVOUS	OVERWHELMED
PEACEFUL	PROUD	RELIEVED
RESENTFUL	SAD	SATISFIED
SCARED	SHOCKED	SELF CONSCIOUS
SILLY	STUPID	SUSPICIOUS
TENSE	TERRIFIED	TRAPPED
WORRIED	WORTHLESS	UNCOMFORTABLE

Chapter Four

Stay Present

It's just a matter of time.

I've always had a tricky relationship with time. In my drinking days, I would lose it in the haze of the evening and try to coax it back in the morning when I'd wake up with a screaming hangover, longing for that extra hour of sleep. It was never on my side and we were constantly at odds.

It didn't help matters that I was living in the past. I was struggling to get over a relationship that had created a tailspin of pain and guilt that wouldn't leave my side for several years. The more I drank, the more warped and out of proportion my memories of it became. Especially the good ones. Leaving the toxicity and dysfunction of my experience behind and painting a picture of 100% tranquility that simply wasn't there.

Time can really do a number on us as we develop habits around how we perceive it. Depending on the course our lives have taken, it can create a preoccupation with either the past or the future, leaving us distracted from the real objective, which is to live our lives in the present.

It's known that emotional maturity is typically stalled at the age we began our addiction. So, for those of us who started drinking heavily in our late teens or early 20s, and got sober in our 30s or 40s, we are far more susceptible to attaching to a time in the past. This is our safe place. It is what's familiar, but it keeps us from moving forward and we end up avoiding having to face a present we aren't yet equipped to face.

In our time travel, we typically fall into one of three categories. Past Focused, Present Focused, or Future Focused and each one of these can take on a negative or positive tone. This becomes a preferred reference point we gravitate toward when thinking about our lives.

Past Focused

If you're Past Focused, you tend to stay stuck in a moment or period of time gone by. This could be in relationship with ourselves or another person, the way we perceived our childhood in general, or simply a moment captured in our memory that is a constant in our mind. Since these can have positive or negative overtones, one is typically predominant.

If you're *positive past focused*, you may love to think back on your glory days as the most popular girl at school or high school track star. Although these may be fond memories, staying invested in those days of grandeur when you were in your "heyday" can keep you from moving on and creating other positive experiences in your life.

If you're *negative past focused*, you may continue to think back on how you were always a C student or never felt loved as a child, which can bring about feelings of inadequacy or being unlovable. Holding onto past resentments or anger can create a stalled state of being that doesn't serve. Staying invested in your perception of the past can distract you from creating meaningful relationships in the here and now.

Future Focused

If you're *positive future focused*, you could be the insatiable optimist or the one who's always waiting for your ship to come in. Stock brokers are a good example of this, always betting on the future. This tends to take the practicality out of the picture, rocking stability and can cause a roller coaster existence.

If you're *negative future focused*, you have a tendency to look at the future as gloom and doom and are hyper focused on the "what ifs." This alarmist attitude has its obvious drawbacks, with the potential to cause depression and a whole host of other health issues.

Present Focused

If you're *positive present focused*, you are constantly looking for the charge in each moment. Partiers and dare devils fall into this category. Filling life up with attempts to keep things lively and carefree. The risk is when you're constantly preoccupied with chasing the thrill, you tend to neglect the nuance in your life. This typically leads to disappointment and a lack of engagement when things aren't running at high speed.

If you're *negative present focused*, you see reality as a disappointment. If you fall into this category, you're typically very sad, angry, or looking at the glass half empty in your approach to life. This is in most cases a disproportionate reaction to what is happening moment by moment. As you apply this negative filter on your daily experiences, it puts you in a constant fog, drowning out any positive aspects that come into play. This consistent outlook can also lead to depression or other health issues.

As you can see, there are many different ways to slice it and the choice is literally up to you.

Your Story

Our relationship with time, whether it's negative or positive, past, present, or future, is shaped by our thoughts and becomes our core focal point. The truth is that it's nothing more than a story we create in our heads. This story is based on thoughts we have that form our beliefs. In order to shift our focus back to the present, we need to identify this story and begin to dismantle it.

For example, if you had a failed romantic relationship in college and you carried that story of failure forward to today, your perception of the past leads you to believe that you're unsuccessful in relationships. Using that reference point as the lens you put on all of your intimate relationships moving forward. Can you see how limiting that can be? You could carry that belief through many years without realizing that you have a disproportionate attachment to a situation that occurred in your past, and if not checked, could shape the outcome of your relationships for years to come.

The Grey

The ultimate goal is to invest in the present moment with a realistic perspective rooted in reality. Overextending one way or another can lead to a heightened sense of either good or bad, which is not ideal.

Before we stopped drinking, there's a tendency for us to see either black or white. More often than not, we were either feeling satisfied with something or seeing red. This is a trick our brain played on us and is in direct correlation to having a toxic substance in our system on a consistent basis, calling the shots. Our goal in recovery is to get back to the grey. That is a more nuanced approach to life and takes into consideration all sides, allowing us to arrive at a more informed conclusion.

The place of understanding where there are positive circumstances as well as negative ones affecting the outcomes in our lives is where we want to be. As long as we keep our lives in perspective, we have a far greater chance of succeeding in recovery.

The good news is that when we enter recovery, time becomes more precious, because once we break free of our addiction and have more substance to fill up our days, we realize that we don't have much of it to waste.

This is why it's so critical to understand where your focus lies. Are you pre-occupied with what has happened or what is yet to come? Staying in the present time keeps us connected to what's happening around us, owning our sobriety, and contributing to the here and now.

When those tendencies to deny our reality arise, perhaps to avoid conflict or discomfort, it's important for us to bring ourselves back into the moment. Time is our teacher and it's critical to our sustained recovery to keep it in perspective.

The BS

The present is too difficult. It's much easier for me to relive the past because that's when I felt true happiness. That feeling can't be replicated. It was good and then everything changed for me. I have no way of going back, so I'm better off keeping my memories close by my side.

Blockers

The blocker here is actually you. There is a reason we try to distract ourselves from the here and now. We need to call ourselves out of living in a different time zone and bring ourselves back to the present, where the real work needs to happen.

You may also have individuals in your life who like to remind you of your past for their own reasons, but it's entirely up to you to keep focused and change that at any given moment.

The Shift

Living in the present is what's important to me. The moment I step out of this frame I go into thoughts and behaviors that are not grounded in reality. Keeping my attention on what is happening on a minute-by-minute basis allows me to face my challenges and not escape them. The greatest gift I can give myself is my willingness to fully participate in my life, appreciate what is and address the ups and downs head on.

Daily Practice

Start recognizing in your conversation as well as action what you gravitate toward. Do you often think of times gone by or are you an insatiable optimist? Knowing where you fall is all the thought you need to put into it. Acknowledge without judgment. Write it down.

Do you have a tendency to look backward or forward? Once you determine where a majority of your focus lies you can determine what needs to happen to change it. Typically, it's merely catching yourself and deciding to redirect your focus.

Breathing is a great way to bring yourself back into the present moment at any given time. Find a daily meditation that works for you. It doesn't need to be extensive—just a few moments of pause during your day will help you focus on staying grounded and present.

Chapter Five

Crush the Bubble
Keep the thoughts that serve. Lose the rest.

When I decided to run the NYC marathon, I had no running experience. The seed was planted on an unseasonably warm April afternoon as I sat outside on a patio in the West Village sipping cocktails with a few co-workers. Someone brought up the race date and said "Wouldn't it be great if we could see all 5 boroughs in one afternoon?" Having had a fascination with New York since I was young, that was all it took, I was all in.

From that moment forward, I thought to myself, *I am going to do this*. I can remember distinctly, even as the others eventually backed out, believing in my heart that it was my race to run. I was still drinking at the time and the physical challenge probably meant more to me than I realized, but my mind was made up.

My friend Becky joined me after a bit of coaxing and a lot of laughs thinking about what we were actually getting ourselves into. After a few months of training and nothing more than the will to make it happen, we spent the entire day running that race. We certainly didn't set any records (can anyone say "beat the sweep?") but we did what we set out to do. We finished. It was hands down one of the most incredible experiences of my life.

Choice

Without even recognizing it, keeping the consistent thought that it was going to happen, simply made it so. What we don't realize is that we take our thoughts for granted. They have an incredible power over the outcomes in our lives and we tend to pick them randomly based on our mood or what we see as our perspective at the time. What we fail to see is if we were more purposeful and chose them more selectively, we could begin to use them to our advantage and avoid picking the ones that cause us pain.

We spend a majority of our time thinking a certain way and finding evidence to prove it to be true. Can you think of a time when you thought you couldn't accomplish something and it didn't happen? It actually becomes a self-fulfilling prophecy.

We make our minds up about something and then set the wheels in motion to make it so. We have the ability to set ourselves up on a course of success or failure, every time we pick a thought. This is true in every aspect of our lives.

In AA, the familiar saying "your best thinking got you here," tells us that there is work to be done to unravel the thoughts that transported us to this state in the first place. We're here because we left our thoughts unattended and our minds have become a very dangerous place.

In recovery, we come to the party with a whole host of baggage about what we think of ourselves and others, and at times our thoughts are all over the map. We face the challenge of reconstructing these thoughts to create different outcomes.

Inner Voice

We all have a voice inside that can drive a negative state of mind. It is the naysayer or judger in us that has been with us since we were born. In some circles this destructive little whisper is known as our "gremlin."

In the book, *Taming your Gremlin* by Rick Carson, he refers to it in masculine terms and describes it more specifically:

"He uses some of your past experiences to hypnotize you into forming and living your life in accordance with self-limiting and sometimes frightening generalizations about you and what existence holds for you. He wants you to feel bad."

Can you imagine the visual of such a presence in our minds? I see a big burly blob, that is always lurking in the background and orchestrating the instruments in my head. I see mine as feminine and she's the one who keeps me up at night with anxiety over everything and anything, pushing me into a corner of fear, causing me to doubt my ability to handle anything.

Now that I recognize her existence and have an image of her, I'm able to stop her in her tracks and start observing what's happening in the moment. Being in a place of observation neutralizes how I process the thoughts as they enter my mind and I can look at them more objectively. This helps me to pause and make a conscious decision whether or not those thoughts actually serve me. If not, I know I can turn them around.

The Model

Thought work is particularly critical in recovery. It is one of the most impactful ways you can improve your state of mind, and once you have the hang of it, it can happen quite quickly. Listening to your thoughts provides essential insight into how you view the world. Your thoughts are a big deal. They not only form your belief system, but they direct the way you feel emotionally and ultimately the circumstances in your life.

I've had the good fortune to work with a brilliant life coach, Brooke Castillo, over the past several years and she introduced me to her ground breaking Thought Model that's incredibly powerful and literally transformed the way I look at my mind and my ability to create the outcomes in my life. The model essentially assesses five interrelated components in our lives: circumstances, thoughts, feelings, actions, and results. Let's break this down a bit further:

Circumstances are the things that are outside of our control. This could be other people, our past, or the weather. Circumstances can essentially be proven in the court of law. As in "I have kids" or "it's 53 degrees outside."

Keep in mind, you may have thoughts about these circumstances, but that is not the factual data.

Thoughts are the sentences that run through our heads when we put meaning to circumstances. We choose these thoughts every day. As in "My kids are stubborn" or "it's way too cold outside."

Keep in mind, the way you frame your thoughts is a choice. You can think negatively or positively about any circumstance. It is entirely up to you.

Feelings are the emotions or vibrations we experience in our body and they are directly related to our thoughts. Examples could be anger, happiness, or sadness resulting from having a certain thought. These are voluntary because we can actually change our emotions when we change our thoughts.

Keep in mind, if you want to change the way you feel about anything, change the way you think about it.

Actions refer to behavior, reaction, or inaction and they are directly related to our feelings. An example would be drinking a bottle of wine because we are feeling lonely, or withdrawing from relationships because we are feeling angry. Sometimes actions can also be subtle, like a change in the tone of our voice.

Keep in mind, the actions you take are merely a response to either a positive or negative feeling.

Results are the direct effect of our actions. This could be gaining weight or a distant relationship with a friend.

Keep in mind, the results you create in your life are the final step in a chain reaction that was started by a thought.

These different components work very closely together. Your circumstances can trigger your thoughts, at which point the domino effect occurs. Your thoughts cause your feelings, your feelings cause the actions you take. and your actions cause the results in your life. You see how that works? The great news is that your thoughts are the linchpin to everything AND you are totally in control of what you decide to think every moment of every day. How awesome is that?

The real magic happens with your thoughts. They will determine how you feel about every aspect of your life and managing them is the key to shifting the outcome. So, when you put this into action you can take any thought you have and run it through the model. Let's give a simple example of the model in action to show you how this works:

Circumstance—A speaking engagement
Thought—I am not a good public speaker
Feeling—fear, anxiety
Action—you don't prepare for the speech
Result—your speech doesn't go well

In this example, you end up creating the evidence to support your thought. Your thought is that you are incapable, which makes you feel fear and anxiety. This causes you to give up and not prepare, leaving the inevitable outcome of bombing your presentation. Your action that was brought on by the emotion you created actually ends up proving that thought. Now, let's turn this around:

Circumstance—A speaking engagement
Thought—I have something important to say
Feeling—confidence, excitement
Action—you dive into preparing for the speech
Result—your speech is a success

Do you see how this works? The way you think about it has created a feeling of confidence and excitement which sets off a whole different chain reaction. You take action according to how you feel. In this case, you are eager to dive in and with preparation comes success!

Let's try one more that may be a bit more relevant to us:

Circumstance—I don't drink

Thought—I don't fit in

Feeling—sadness, anger, loneliness

Action—you withdraw and become anti-social

Result—you are lonely and don't give yourself a chance to fit in.

Thinking that you don't fit in is in effect causing you to create that reality. The way you frame your thoughts are directly related to how you feel. This reaction then sets you on either a positive or negative course. It's entirely up to you. The way to reframe it would be:

Circumstance—I don't drink.

Thought—I'm so fortunate to be sober

Feeling—calm, grateful

Action—you seek out others with similar experience

Result—you build a supportive community around you.

You are simply one decision away every time. To go with the thought that serves or the one that causes pain.

These are just a few ways to work the model, but you can begin to see how your thoughts are the catalyst for either joy or suffering. Your choice.

This is an amazing tool to use on a daily basis because we all know that our thoughts are swimming around our head constantly. The key is knowing that a) you have a choice to think any thought you want, and b) thoughts have the power to change everything.

I do a significant amount of work with this model in my coaching practice because in recovery we have thoughts that have been with us for years. It takes time to unravel them. Thoughts like, *I'm a failure, I'm not confident, I'm different* are not only harmful to our psyche but they begin to form a belief system that is extremely detrimental to our well-being and can literally unravel our sobriety.

The crazy thing about it is that our thought process is so automatic that many of us are sabotaging our own happiness by crowding our minds with these subtle little buzz kills every minute of every day, and have no idea we're even doing it.

Practicing thought work is the single most precious gift you can give yourself. It allows you to take back the control of how you think about the circumstances in your life and your own personal capabilities.

If you're interested in going deeper into this work, please don't hesitate to reach out to me at noelle@sobermoxie.com and we can talk further about how you can put this into daily practice and become a master of your own mind management.

The BS

My thoughts are a direct result of what has happened to me. I can't help but think the way I do. I am not even in control of them. I don't have a choice. If only she wasn't such a b***, I would think about her differently.

Blockers

Your thoughts can be your best friends or your worst enemies. Letting them control you instead of having a strategy to manage them can be a complete disaster. You are totally in the driver's seat and yet, you tend to spend a great deal of time trying to justify your thoughts rather than recognize that the ones you form are creating your reality. Spending a bit of time with the model will reveal this very clearly.

The Shift

I am the master of my own mind. I have control over feeling good or bad at all times. It's a big responsibility taking accountability for how I feel, but it's worth it. I need to stop hiding behind my thoughts and realize they can be wiggled and changed. This knowledge alone makes it possible for me to create my own outcomes.

Daily Practice

Write down a description of your gremlin. What does it look like? Does it have a name? Personalizing this character in your mind helps you recognize it better when it starts crowding your mind and creating negative thoughts. It gives you more of a chance to calm the gremlin down and put it back in its place as you politely decline the invitation.

I cannot overemphasize the importance of writing down your thoughts. A daily thought download is critical to start getting inside the chatter and examining it.

When you take a closer look at what is lurking around in your head on a daily basis, you're able to decide if it's serving you or not. This exercise, although it may feel tedious, will give you a good indication of what's going on at a deeper level.

The easiest place to start is in the morning. Jotting down what pops into your head when you first wake up is extremely telling. Once you have the thoughts on paper, run them through the model. Doing this on a consistent basis will seriously alter how you process everything that gets thrown in your path. It is really quite amazing.

Some of us wake up anxious about the day ahead, others excited. You will start to make the connection between your thoughts and the vibrations you are experiencing in your body. This leaves it up to you to change them at any given moment. The power is literally in your hands. It's up to you to determine what you are going to do with it.

Chapter Six

Sing Mama Sing!

Let your voice be heard.

I could hear the Howler monkeys outside my window as I drew the curtain open to face another beautiful day in Costa Rica. It was our last day at Blue Spirit for a Recovery 2.0 yoga retreat. I'd been to this magical place several times before and every time I came back, I could see another part of myself a bit more clearly. It has a tendency to lovingly rattle your cage before releasing you back out into the world to put what you've learned into practice.

51

One of the daily rituals for these retreats is to open the day at 6 a.m. with a Sadhana, or spiritual practice, followed by a session in a similar format as a 12 step meeting. I was still feeling a bit conflicted as I went into the final morning practice. Although they say sharing is optional, I was one of a handful of people who hadn't done so yet and this morning I felt a subtle disappointment in myself that seemed to come out of nowhere.

For me, telling my story has always been difficult. I tend to convince myself that I'm just waiting until I have something relevant to say, but I know if I look under the hood, that's merely a delay tactic and excuse to hold back, instead of opening up and speaking from my heart. That's actually never been my forte, to say the least, and something I've grappled with for years.

As the meeting started to come to a close and they asked if anyone had a burning desire to speak, a remarkable thing happened. As if in a trance, I stood up, walked across the room and grabbed the microphone. Some unexplained energy (*aha! there goes that force again*) put my feet into motion well before my brain caught up with what was even happening. I spoke for several minutes and although I don't have exact recall of what I actually said or how I said it, I know it was from the heart.

That's how this crazy thing works. The more in sync we become with our unconscious intention, moments start to pop up where we suddenly get out of our own way. I knew as I sat back down that something had changed. The little voice inside me that wanted to share and connect was taking control and guiding me. I'd overcome my instinct to hide in the shadows and my need to be heard took hold.

Letting ourselves go with this instinct is so important, because although it may be tucked away in the corner of our soul, it's still there. We know deep inside that what we have to offer is important. Even if our ego is trying to tell us otherwise. We must resist the urge to give into it because when we do, everyone loses.

Slow Learner

Needless to say, I was a slow learner when it came to finding my voice. I always knew I had it in me, but I'd suppressed it for so long that I had to take those baby steps to gain the confidence to start putting it back into practice.

Truth be told, I was a pretty excitable child. My family would actually say I was a bit of a hellion. I was the youngest of four and spent the better part of my early childhood stomping my feet, slamming doors and throwing brushes across the room at my sister. I was easy to upset and often found sobbing in my room.

My angst took shape in many ways during my grade school years and I acted out quite a bit. I think the more my behavior disappointed those around me, the more isolated and alone I felt, eventually causing me to rethink my rebellious ways and opt for a more agreeable approach. Little did I know at the time, that this would come at a cost. I began to stuff down my feelings of fear and anger and replaced them with silence and lock jaw acceptance.

My lack of expression was a learned behavior. Somewhere along the way in my mind, speaking my truth seemed to cause disruptive outcomes, so I did as any young unassuming child would do, I shut down my feelings completely and for the next few decades of my life embarked on my own personal crusade of self-censorship.

In my early twenties I sought out relationships with guys who had a similar inability to access their feelings. We were in good company, each of us in our own state of dissociation. They were either alcoholic, emotionally absent, or both. This only reinforced my habit of keeping things locked away. These experiences, along with my growing insecurity, reinforced my belief that having an opinion or voicing my feelings just simply wasn't important.

The Turning Point

After a few years of sobriety, emotions began to show up in odd ways and I knew that my voice could no longer be ignored. As I've participated in the recovery community over the past several years, it's become obvious that I'm not alone.

Some of us experience an inability to speak up and voice our needs or opinions even under the best of circumstances. So, for those of us in recovery, the issue is magnified. We are finally experiencing emotion again and this suppression no longer fits into the mold as our desire increases to live in truth and transparency. We become at odds with what we've learned in the past and what our hearts are telling us to do in the present. This only leads to further negative thinking and anxiety, virtually stalling our healing process.

The good news is as you grow in your sobriety and your voice begins to stir and hum, you can no longer ignore it. It begs for your attention and its whisper grows in intensity, telling you it can no longer be ignored. This is the time to take a leap of faith that will ultimately propel you forward. Recovery calls on you to reconnect with feelings and express your truth, desires, and opinions in a healthy way. It just takes time and willingness to get there.

One of my clients had always struggled to find her voice around her mother. After further examination she realized that the lack of connection between them was due to her mother's co-dependency with her brother who had fallen deeper into his addiction over the years. We worked together to take a closer look at the belief system her mom had developed in response to the devastation of her brother's situation. In doing so, she was able to reframe the messaging and look at her mother's distance with compassion and greater objectivity. Once she was able to accept it as her mother's experience, not her own, she was able to break free and liberate herself to speak her truth.

It's critical now more than ever to listen to your inner truth and express it without reservation. Until you do, you'll remain stuck and unable to open up and fully experience the miracles that are waiting to unfold in your life.

Expressing yourself can be exceptionally challenging. Especially if you've spent a significant amount of time drinking to numb out and shut down your emotions. You've learned to build up a resistance to expression over time. It either started at a young age or developed gradually and may have been brought on by trauma or relationships that reinforced the behavior of staying quiet and shut down. Regardless of how you learned it, the desire to hold back your feelings at some point became a means of survival.

It's no wonder that when you get sober and begin to explore a deeper relationship with yourself that you seem stuck and ill equipped to know how you feel let alone how to express it. The desire to change is the first step. Voice can be recognized in many different ways. All it takes is recognition of your truth, developing your conviction, and practice, practice, practice.

Risk

It's easy for us to become very self-absorbed in recovery. We think that our reality of feeling separate and alone is unique. The truth is that a majority of the population, sober or not, experience their share of self-doubt and fear when speaking their truth. In a way, it's very selfish to worry about what others think of our thoughts, feelings, or opinions. It keeps the spotlight shining inward rather than focusing on a commitment to creating deeper connection with others.

Once we reframe it and look at it as a means of relaying information that will broaden perspective and help others better understand a different point of view, it lessens the perceived personal risk and opens us up to doing it more often.

I ask my clients to think about it this way; if you were in a situation where a loved one was being held hostage and you had to negotiate with the captors, but the only way you could do it was through a microphone, in front of a room full of people, would you shy away, or think twice of what they thought of you? Of course not.

In this example, you are laser focused on the objective of bringing your loved one to safety and would do whatever it took to achieve it. Right? The "you" in the equation fades away and your voice becomes the messenger, there to relay important information needed to achieve an outcome.

Although it may seem counterintuitive, perceived risk tends to decrease when there's more at stake. It fades into the background when the consequences of not expressing yourself become detrimental. You need to start thinking of your participation in the larger dialog of life as joining the big league. Everything you do from now on is paving the way for you to become a bolder, stronger player in the game. Without it, you are merely sitting on the sidelines letting others have the conversation and deciding for you how you will experience your life.

One of the commitments you made in recovery was to stop drinking. That was merely removing the obstacle that kept you quiet in the first place. What are you going to do with your new found gift? Now it's time to bring forth what the world needs to hear.

Start participating. Speak up and be heard.

The BS

I have nothing important to say. Speaking up only makes me feel uncomfortable and no one cares about what I have to say anyway. My opinion won't make a difference. I've always been quiet. I'm not like most people who just like to hear themselves talk.

Blockers

There will always be someone else who will step up when you decide to back down. It is up to you to give yourself permission to take the first step and commit to it. Once that happens, the next time will only become easier. When expressing yourself, the key to success is practice. That means risking potential failure in order to overcome your habit of hiding. It also means accepting the invitation to do so, time and again.

The Shift

The world is waiting to hear from me. The avoidance game is over. It's time for me to be seen and heard and felt by others. Staying in close connection with my emotions is the key to expressing myself in the moment. Showing up in a strong and confident way is a key milestone in recovery. It tells the world I am ready for more. No one else can bring this forth but me.

Daily Practice

Sing Mama Sing! Yep, that's what I said. It's time to start singing. Wherever, whenever, and as often as you can. Even if you're horrible, that's just fine. No one even needs to hear you. Sing in the shower, in the car, to your dog, to your baby. It will loosen up your vocal cords and break down your inhibition the more you practice.

Start listing the areas in your life where your voice is quieted—either by yourself or others. How can you shift that dynamic? What is holding you back? Is it other people's agenda you are living by?

Make a commitment to express your opinion in some way big or small to others, at every chance you get. You can start out on social media to ease in. Facebook is a great example of a forum to use to get the word out on topics you want to talk about or endorse. Then take the steps toward doing so in one-on-one conversations. Whatever works for you, start forming the habit of expressing yourself, and soon it will be easier to do without reservation. As in song, the experience of hearing yourself speak is a very valuable one. The auditory playback is very powerful.

Lastly, find something blue to wear around your neck. It can be a necklace or a scarf. The color blue supports the throat chakra and is a wonderful way to remind yourself of your need to consistently speak up.

Chapter Seven

Breathe
Mindfulness is magic.

I made my way into my naturopath's office knowing I was late. I'd scheduled this appointment as a routine check in. I'd been feeling out of sorts for a while so she recommended I do a blood panel and a few tests to make sure everything was normal and to check my hormone levels. I received my results at my last visit and all looked good, so I expected this would be a quick follow up for me to give her an update, pick up a refill or two, and be on my way. What I didn't realize was that the results of my adrenal test had just arrived.

As we sat down at her desk, she looked a bit cautious and began to run through my numbers. I think she could see the confused look on my face, and decided to cut to the chase because she paused for a moment and then asked "Have you ever heard of severe adrenal fatigue?"

I stumbled to come up with a response. I didn't have a clue what adrenal fatigue was and hearing that mine was apparently severe made me a bit nervous. She could see I was baffled and began to describe the correlation between high stress, alcoholism, and adrenal gland overload, and suddenly the pieces began to fall into place.

Looking back, I realized I'd been fighting stress and anxiety most of my adult life. I picked a profession in HR that put me right in the mix of high pressure start-up environments, and when I think of my general disposition, although I can be pretty calm on the outside, my co-dependent tendencies often caused me to take on other people's drama and energy along with my own—overloading me at times with unnecessary worry. I laughed to myself thinking, *there couldn't have been a more perfect storm of factors in my life to lead me to this.*

In addition to high stress, she began to unravel the harm alcohol addiction does to the central nervous system, and how it puts our adrenals into a state of complete overload in the process. She explained that the nervous system is the set of circuitry that allows our body to take on the blows of the outside world and acts as an internal regulator that keeps us in balance. They drive our fight or flight response and once they become over taxed, their functioning can be compromised. This can cause a bunch of potential problems that can include anxiety, and you guessed it, severe adrenal fatigue.

I find it ironic that we drink to relax, and in the process we deplete our body's natural ability to bring us back to that state, only increasing our feeling of dis-ease and discomfort. A hamster wheel situation if there ever was one. With these cards stacked against us, it's a sure bet that once we get sober there's a bit of rebalancing that needs to be done.

Needless to say, this new realization and strict orders to lower my stress levels only deepened my resolve to maintain better balance. After trying many different methods of relaxation from sauna to massage to Reike, I finally landed on one of the most highly underrated means of reaching a state of natural calm. Reconnecting with my breath.

Breathe

If you've ever had a panic attack, you know what it's like to be disconnected with your breath. As you gasp for air and your heart starts racing you can feel your body in a state of heightened agitation.

What most sober people don't know is that with the exception of those who suffer from mental illnesses (also known as co-addictions), for many of us, learning to breathe properly can significantly reduce our anxiety and exponentially increase our ability to sustain our sobriety.

As we all know, entering recovery can be very disorienting. Especially in the beginning, you're stumbling your way through a fun house of trap doors and mazes trying to find some semblance of peace and calm. As your cells begin to repair, sensation comes back again, in full force. This is why when we first get sober, some of us feel exceptionally raw and sensitive to outside stimuli. Our senses are returning and the influx of inputs feels overwhelming.

I tell people all the time that the best way to get your bearings and start to feel grounded is to get comfortable with silence and listening to your body. By that I mean, be aware of what's going on and learn techniques to bring yourself back to a calm and relaxed state at any given moment.

This is the time where finding our breath becomes most important. Learning to breathe properly can literally alter the systems within our body allowing us to naturally heal. I sought out yoga to become more in tune with my body and as I stumbled upon the practice of kundalini, it opened my eyes to the miracle of breath work.

Breath of Fire

Breath of Fire was first taught to me at a kundalini yoga retreat. It's a rhythmic breath with equal emphasis on the inhale and exhale, no deeper than sniffing. It's done by pumping the naval point towards the spine on the exhale and releasing the naval out on the inhale. It's practiced through the nostrils with your mouth and eyes closed. When done correctly, you should feel as if you can go indefinitely.

In addition to resetting your sympathetic and parasympathetic nervous system, other benefits of Breath of Fire range from massaging your internal organs to purifying the blood and releasing deposits from the lungs. Circulating oxygen through the body in this way also stimulates the solar plexus, generating heat and releasing natural energy throughout the body.

Using this technique is the first step in using breath as a tool to support our natural healing process. It is an amazing exercise that practiced on a regular basis can have a remarkable effect on your state of well-being.

Mindfulness

Meditation is an effective way to slow down our bodies and minds and look inward. Pacing our breath can be very beneficial in pausing, reflecting, and even reaching a state of deep inner peace. It's a powerful way to connect with ourselves and we can reach this state simply by following the rhythm of our inhale and exhale.

When you think of meditation, you may think of a guru sitting on a pillow, chanting in the corner of some dark and cavernous monastery. Although that may be the scene in some parts of the world, the truth is, any form of quiet can be considered meditation. It can be done on the floor of your living room, on your mat or even while out on a walk. It's simply a state of relaxation that brings peace and awareness to your consciousness at any given moment. It is in this space where we can cut out the noise, plug in, and be truly mindful.

Mindfulness Based Stress Reduction (MBSR) was developed back in the '70s by Dr. Jon Kabat-Zinn, at the UMASS Medical Center/Stress-Reduction Clinic and Center for Mindfulness. It was set up to help assist people with pain and a range of conditions and life issues that were initially difficult to treat in a hospital setting.

This is what I consider to be the mac daddy of programs for those looking to incorporate all elements of mindfulness into their daily practice. It consists of learning, practicing, and integrating the various methods of mindfulness. This includes body scanning and different elements of yoga and meditation.

I was turned onto this practice a while back by a friend and teacher of mine, Cassie Schindler, who is an exceptional meditation and mindfulness guide. I was struck at how much this consistent practice can help not only in maintaining a healthy lifestyle but also in addressing chronic pain and anxiety. It's become more mainstream over the years and is now taught in hospitals around the world. It's also starting to catch on in corporate America to help decrease work related stress.

Regardless of how shallow or deep you go with this, it is safe to say that incorporating a mechanism to slow down, breathe deeply, and become mindful of what is happening around you will do wonders for your state of mind and body.

The BS

I have no idea how to meditate and can't sit still for any period of time. I don't understand it and I think doing breathing exercises is a bunch of bunk. I need to learn to calm down on my own. Yoga just isn't going to do it for me.

Blockers

Once you start telling people you are doing Breath of Fire every morning, get ready for a few blank stares. People who don't get it aren't meant to! They are not here to approve your actions and you are not here to seek their approval. In fact, I would advise you to not try to convert your mother or husband for that matter if they are considered more conservative in their approach to healing. As we have come to learn, sometimes sharing too much with others who are not on the same path can run the risk of discouraging you from trying a powerful technique that can make a true difference in your life.

The Shift

Learning to self soothe is critical in my recovery. Meditation and breath work may seem unconventional, but they truly work for me. Breath work is one of the most powerful methods of healing and the great news is—it's absolutely free! I incorporate these practices into my daily routine because they bring me back to a state of balance, and I understand the connection between deep relaxation and optimum health.

Daily Practice

Three minutes of Breath of Fire every morning can change your life! Set your timer, in a seated position, hold your fingers bent at the knuckles with your thumbs tucked in. Raise your arms above your head, shoulder width apart and begin to inhale and exhale as stated above. Remember to release your belly on the inhale and bring it toward your spine on the exhale. Make sure to bring in an equal amount of air on the inhale and exhale as well. Otherwise, you may feel a bit light headed. As you close your eyes, focus your internal gaze on the third eye which is the point between your eyes. Sit in silence for a few minutes as you draw the energy up within your body. You will begin to notice a change in your overall state almost immediately. Try doing this for 30 days in a row and you'll feel the difference.

Find a place and a time for meditation that is away from your usual routine. It could be in a room in your house, in your yard, or on your yoga mat. Anywhere you feel comfortable and can get away from the noise of life.

Chapter Eight

Take Care

You owe it to yourself and others.

It was a cold November morning as I stood in line outside of a little theatre on the upper west side waiting to be let into my first workshop with the Institute for Integrative Nutrition. I was more than eager to get started. I had spent most of my time gobbling up books on nutrition and I was fascinated by all of the different philosophies there were out there on how best to fuel the body. I was ironically well into my addiction by then and fighting a physical war with myself on a daily basis, which in hindsight must have been fueling my curiosity.

Learning about nutrition and going on to receive my certification as a health coach only strengthened my conviction that when provided with the right nutrients, the body has a natural way of bringing itself back into balance.

As they say, our body is a temple. In our addiction, we treat our body more like a dumping ground, overloading it with toxic substances, lack of sleep, and self- induced stress. As we make our way into recovery, our bodies are bouncing back as best as they can, but it takes time and attention to restore ourselves back to health.

I may start sounding like a broken record here, but it all comes back to balance. Finding this in general can be a huge challenge. As women, we are programmed to multi-task and take care of others at our own expense. This, as we know, is a recipe for disaster. Knowing that we are so much more alert and alive when we feel rested and nourished, it is of utmost importance for us to listen to our own needs and take the time to practice self-care. Without it, we are doing ourselves as well as our loved ones a disservice.

Healing from addiction is a process and eating right to get your body back on track is extremely important. There are some critical components to a diet targeted at replenishing the body especially when it's in need of repair.

I could drone on for hours about this topic but I want to stay focused on the basics here because all it takes is a few key shifts in how you nourish your body that can make all the difference in the world. So, I am going to break it down into three critical components: nutrition, movement, and elimination.

Nutrition

Always start by focusing on foods that will help replace lost nutrients. Since alcohol tends to deplete your body of large quantities of vitamins and minerals, replenishing these are your first step in recovery. Thiamine, B-6, and folate are the biggies, so you should incorporate them into your daily diet as your body doesn't easily store them.

Good sources of thiamine include vegetables, fruit, eggs, and whole-grain bread. Vitamin B-6 is found in pork, poultry, and fish in addition to many of the sources of thiamine. Folate can be found in many green vegetables, like broccoli, spinach, or peas.

A nutrient-dense diet rich in B vitamins, organic protein, plenty of leafy greens and vegetables, low-sugar fruits, and a variety of healthy, healing fats is the best diet for a recovering alcoholic. Protein and fat in particular help prevent blood sugar fluctuations, increase energy, fuel the brain, and eliminate cravings.

Women should also take calcium as part of their daily supplements since heavy drinking increases the risk of osteoporosis. Even women who don't drink are at much higher risk than men for this bone-weakening disease. I know, lucky us!

<u>Sugar</u>
Blood sugar fluctuations can happen frequently once you stop drinking. Since alcohol has such a high sugar content, once it's eliminated from your diet, your tendency may be to look for substitutes like candy or pastries to curb your cravings, causing these levels to spike and dip repeatedly.

I often recommend raw honey or stevia when looking for a good sugar substitute. They are low in calories, don't spike sugar levels, and make a huge difference in satisfying a sweet tooth.

Sugar is a trap that many of us can fall into if we're not careful. Alcoholics have a predisposition to sugar sensitivities in the first place, so once it's taken away, our cravings can go through the roof and we end up replacing one addiction for another.

I've found that the best way to counteract this is to eat snacks with protein or fruit high in fiber such as apples or pears, coupled with a healthy fat. Almond and peanut butter are some of my favorites.

I've had issues with hypoglycemia all my life and have always balanced carbs with protein and healthy fats. If my first meal of the day contains all three, it sets me up with more consistent energy throughout the day.

Healthy Fats

Healthy fats are also something to keep in our diets. The fats found in omega-3 and omega-6 fatty acids have multiple health benefits and can help everything from pain management and bone health to decreasing inflammation. Inflammation in the joints and muscles in particular can be caused by alcohol use, so including healthy oils in on your daily menu is a good idea. I personally love Udo's Oil 3-6-9 Blend. It provides all the fatty acids in one fell swoop and is easy to throw in smoothies or on a salad.

Antioxidants

Finally, antioxidants help to fight free radicals in the body. Especially for those who have had a long history of alcohol use, who could be susceptible to liver damage, eating foods with antioxidants can help to improve and support ongoing health. Foods high in antioxidants include blueberries, gogi berries, pecans, artichokes, and yes, thankfully dark chocolate! Vitamin C also packs a punch, so taking your daily Cs with your daily Bs is ideal.

I actually have an amazing smoothie that I highly recommend. It's easy to make and is packed with vitamin B, healthy oils, and disease fighting super foods. I call it my Super B Blast! Perfect for any time of the day. If you are interested in trying it out, here's the recipe:

1 cup water
A handful of ice
1 cup of blueberries
1/2 apple
1 cup Kale or Spinach
1/2 cucumber
1 teaspoon Oil (i.e. Udo's Oil 3-6-9 blend)
1 cup powder protein—(ie. Vega one)
Mix it up in the blender and enjoy!

An important thing to remember when changing your diet to support the healing process is to always keep it simple. As we all know, the more complicated the regiment the less likely we are to follow it. That's just typically the deal. So make it easy on yourself and find ways to incorporate foods that matter into no fuss meals.

Movement

I had a huge awakening when I started my yoga practice over 5 years ago. I had actually started "doing" yoga as a form of exercise well before that, but as I learned more about the power of movement in processing emotion and centering myself, it began to have a deeper purpose.

Daily exercise is a huge component of staying healthy and if you've been around long enough, you understand the benefits of incorporating movement into your daily routine. Raising your heart rate is a powerful thing in and of itself, but it has been said that exercise can also help to repair damaged nerve connections within the central nervous system. As we mentioned in the previous chapter, this system is one of the hardest hit by alcohol use.

The misconception we often have is that exercise needs to be high impact in order to be effective. Nothing could be farther from the truth. Low impact activities such as walking, swimming, or practicing yoga can provide just as many health benefits as running, biking, or playing tennis. The important aspect that they all share is moving the body and raising the heart rate.

Keeping our body moving is key and not just for the physical benefits, but mental as well. In a recent book I read called *Waking the Tiger* by Peter A. Levine, he talks about the cycle of trauma and how we hold our experiences in our bodies as well as our minds. It's a fascinating study about animals and their immunity to traumatic symptoms, but it highlights the importance of accessing and resolving past experience in order to fully process the trauma. It's similar to the concept of bringing emotion up and out in order to let it go.

Yoga has the ability to make us physically stronger and more resilient and is a powerful catalyst for this to happen. We can begin to feel the way this works when we are in poses that cause resistance or discomfort. Often times when this happens the power of sitting with the discomfort can help to bring up emotions from the past that may have not been processed and need to be released.

Rest

If you're a night owl, what I'm about to say may sound a little crazy, but 7-8 hours of sleep a night is recommended to receive optimal benefits. Now, I am fully aware that this is my personal sweet spot because I rarely am able to keep my eyes open after 9pm, but it's something worth considering if you are not prone to calling it a day any time before midnight.

Getting enough sleep is so underrated. We tend to downplay the importance of rest because we are a society of "doers" but I'm here to tell you, more rest is a very good thing. I am indirectly speaking to my mom as well who used to be known as the "nap cop" in our house. For years, she showed absolutely no respect for the power of a good ole fashioned mid-day snooze. Banging around to make sure no one was nodding off, the woman was relentless. I'm happy to say now that she's retired, she finally gave in and finds herself nodding off mid-day for an hour or so to recharge. I'd like to say Mom, I think you've officially come over to the dark side.

Sleep can help reduce stress, improve metabolism, and even improve your memory! Having spent a few years coming out of a post alcoholic fog with what felt like a temporary loss of short term recall, this is definitely good news!

Needless to say, if you are able to get to sleep early enough to snag those precious hours of shut eye a night, you will feel a difference and be well ahead of the game.

Elimination

Elimination or gentle detox is important in bringing our bodies back into a healthy state. If I were to think of three key recommendations I would give for supporting this process (along with a healthy diet) they would be probiotics, body brushing, and dry saunas.

Alcohol can do a number on our digestive tract while we are drinking and the damage can remain severe often after we stop. It can disrupt our body's natural balance and in more severe instances, can lead to ulcers or endotoxins to leak into the gut causing what is known as "leaky gut". If you're experiencing pain or discomfort it's best to consult your physician. However, for those of you who are looking to rebalance, probiotics can be hugely beneficial. They not only help to restore your body's ability to fight off disease, but also support regular elimination which is important when experiencing a detox of any kind. You can find probiotics at any health food store. I personally like Ultimate Flora.

Since our skin is our biggest organ, dry body brushing helps awaken the body and sluff off toxins that come to the surface of our skin, particularly during detox. If you are on a detox program or simply starting in recovery, this daily routine right before showering is particularly beneficial. You want to lightly brush over your skin in a sweeping motion. Make sure to cover your body from your toes up to your neck. Always brush toward your heart since this activity stimulates blood circulation. You can purchase a natural brush at any whole foods or bath shop and just hang it in your shower for easy use.

Dry saunas are one of my favorite ways to support natural detox. The heat is relaxing and it stimulates blood flow while eliminating toxins through perspiration. If you are less into dry heat, you can also use a steam room to get a similar effect.

Drinking has put our bodies in a state of dis-ease. We've been thrown off kilter and need to flush toxins out of our body. Elimination is of utmost importance in this detoxification process. The three areas of focus we've discussed in this chapter are only scratching the surface, but if you incorporate them into your daily routine, they can be fundamental in restoring our body back to health.

The BS

I have done so much damage to my body, what's it going to matter if I start paying attention to it now? I'm not sure I want to think so much about my diet. Since I can't drink anymore, I feel like I deserve to indulge in foods that may not be great for me, but make me feel better.

Blockers

Those around us who see us eating better are typically supportive. It's the subtle temptations that sometimes flash before us that can make things difficult. Mom's favorite brownie recipe or your partner's famous Fettuccini Alfredo. All offered with love but can be deadly when we are trying to stay on track. The other blocker can be time. We often find that exercise and diet hit the back burner when time is limited.

The Shift

As I start to get back into balance and become more aware of my body's needs, I am instinctively starting to treat it with more care. I know how years of abuse and neglect have made me feel, and having energy and stamina are so much more important to me now. Caring for my body has become second nature and I am ready to make the time for it.

Daily Practice

Start thinking of movement as a way to bring emotion up and out of your body. Take a longer walk than usual to soak up the scenery. Hold a pose a bit longer than usual. Try to push past the discomfort and make note of how it feels. What does your body want to do? If you are squirming to get out of it, observe and reflect on what your body is trying to tell you. The more you work from a place of non-judgmental observation the more you will learn about what you are still holding onto and what needs to be released.

For those of you who have trouble winding down at night, try "legs up the wall" pose. As the name suggests, just lay on the floor with your legs up the wall. This helps soothe your nervous system and bring your body into deep relaxation. I typically do this for approx. 5-10 minutes before I go to bed at night. When I do, I notice a big difference in how much easier it is to fall asleep and I typically stay down longer.

Keep a food journal. I used to hate these until I took the judgment away. In my quest to cut the sugar (which I continue to battle), it was really telling to see what time of day I was more susceptible to eating poorly. I was like a detective. With this information, I was better prepared for it to happen and began to make wiser food choices to help curb the cravings. Writing it down provides you with the data you need to more successfully disrupt the patterns.

Chapter Nine

Moxie Baby

**Live life on your own terms.
Make them non-negotiable.**

I wish I had some remarkable story about how I took life into my own hands and now live a flawless existence where I confidently do things my way every day. I would be lying if I said that was the case, but I can tell you that I am miles ahead of where I used to be, and I can honestly say that I no longer let others dictate my choices. I let my wants and needs take the lead.

It's a simple equation and it all starts when you make the decision to get sober. If that is not a sign of moving closer to living life on your own terms, I don't know what is. Making that decision actually created a subtle tension between you and a majority of the population who continue to drink. You may have even received flack, not praise, when you went into recovery. Strange as it sounds, most people don't like change. Period. Sometimes even if that change is necessary to save a friend's life. Most people are busy worrying about themselves and you can guarantee that no one experiences life exactly the same way you do, which is all the more reason to call your own shots.

You make the critical choice each and every day to live your life free of alcohol, the one thing that used to make you feel alive. You've foregone the allure of short-term relief for the benefits of a life untethered by the pain and anguish of addiction and that my friend, is HUGE!

Think about it. You've done all of this in the face of unbelievable odds. All in the presence of well assuming friends and family who would do absolutely anything to keep you safe, but if push came to shove, would be virtually unable to stop you if you decided to drink again. That's terrifying for sure, but even more reason to hold your sobriety in your own hands as a fragile and coveted gift that should never, under any circumstances, be taken for granted.

Knowing this, we all have to face the facts that we live in a tipsy world and are in a culture that is dripping with booze. It is virtually everywhere, on billboards, in magazines, on TV, and in the movies. Not to mention around every corner, enticing us to forego sobriety and come out and play. Offering up the quick drink after work, inviting you to the cocktail party, or the happy hour at the cozy little wine bar across the street. Urging you to relax, lighten up, and have a good time with the promise of tucking you in and making life warm and comfortable again.

You are called each and every day to reject the temptation of giving in and joining the masses. Resisting the gentle nudge that beckons you to slide on over and belly up to the bar. But you know better. You know this seductive little glass of heaven is really the devil in disguise. You know that one false move and you'd be right back on a spiral of self-destruction that could easily take you down, for good.

So living life on your own terms in sobriety is not only important, it's essential to your survival. When you finally make the critical decision to call your own shots, it has a domino effect. You start paying closer attention to other areas of your life. This is when the real work begins.

Spring Cleaning
Don't you just love the feeling you get after a good spring cleaning? I'm not talking about a little sweeping up here and

there on the weekend, I'm talking about the sense of satisfaction you get after you've gone to town on your floors and fixtures, done the dusting and hit all of the nooks and crannies that you've neglected over the past several months. Everything feels so new and inviting.

The idea of tidying up when it comes to the people you surround yourself with sounds like a somewhat radical concept, but it's something we all need to do once in a while. Our time is precious and we need to take stock in how we spend it, since being around positive and supportive energy is critical to our success in sustaining our sobriety.

If we think about it, how many years have we spent caring about what others think of us? When we were little, we lived in the moment. We didn't have a clue about what others thought of us. It was not until years of seeking approval from our parents and friends that we began to establish a set of beliefs about ourselves based on whether or not we measured up to other people's expectations. That can be exhausting.

The good news about beliefs is that they are just a bunch of thoughts conjured up in our minds to make up a story and since we now know, they are ultimately ours to choose at any given time, what we believe is completely in our hands.

So, when we decide to determine who we spend our time with, we are making the conscious decision to no longer care what others think of us. That's pretty big stuff. This requires taking a hard look at our existing relationships, nurturing the ones that bring positive energy, and removing the ones that bring negative energy into our lives. This is never an easy task, because as we all know, breaking up is hard to do.

Think of it in terms of energy—you want to avoid surrounding yourself with lower frequencies that could compromise your sobriety. It's time to take a closer look at what needs to change to keep your daily interactions operating at a high frequency. The expectations of others will never go away, so it's up to you to determine how to navigate them when they come into your life. All of our relationships have a time and a purpose, some of them are meant to be short term and others are here for the duration.

The true challenge comes when the people who are not supporting you in a positive way are relatives, especially those who were part of the dance with you when you were drinking. They may be happy you are sober, but not happy with the way it affects their way of life. You may still live with a partner or spouse who continues to drink. This is where boundary setting is critical. You need to establish a new "normal" and bring the folks in your life along with you so they are taught what you will tolerate and what you will not.

In our addiction, boundaries were not our thing. They were virtually non-existent especially for those of us involved in co-dependent relationships where they can become completely blurred. It is as if you don't know where one boundary ends and another begins. For romantic relationships in particular this may cause a mess of unresolved issues that can only amplify once you stop drinking. In recovery, you are called to clean up those tangled webs and start standing on your own two feet, which isn't easy.

It may mean seeking outside relationship guidance for you and your partner or spouse, or lessening time spent in situations that can trigger old behaviors. This could involve threatening the status quo and making new requests to better support your sobriety. Whatever it is, it's a choice you must make for the sake of your own health.

It all starts with identifying what you want to create in your life. Once you understand that, you will know when it's time to weed out the relationships that don't serve and draw in the ones that do.

The BS

My relationship feels strained but I don't want to rock the boat. My partner has been so supportive, I could never ask him to change. I may be unhappy, but I would be miserable without him. I can't go this alone. If I start speaking my mind, he may not love me anymore.

Blockers

Family is often difficult because in some cases, you are stuck with these people for the rest of your life, and in others, making a change could potentially disrupt a way of living you have come to know as safe and comfortable, even if it's not necessarily bringing you happiness. Regardless of the circumstances, sometimes family can be the worst place to look for support. There is a closeness there that takes a healthy perspective out of the equation.

Expectations can be strong and you often revert back to a time when acceptance from your parents was your main objective. This can mess with you, because if the need for approval you sought as a child still hasn't been met, it's most likely not coming your way as an adult either, so it becomes a fruitless pursuit.

The Shift

Having a vision of who I want around me and how I want to show up in my life is invaluable. One actually affects the other. If I surround myself with positivity, my life will begin to change in amazing ways. Support in sobriety is underrated. It is incredibly important to have friends, partners, and family members who are there for me in good times and in bad, and are willing to put themselves aside to embrace the new me.

Daily Practice

Determine what fills you up. What energy is the most important for you to be around? Write it down.

Take a look at your relationships with friends, co-workers, and family. For the ones that aren't working, list the things about those relationships that bring you to a place of depletion. What can you do to improve the ones that need to change? Do the same for relationships that are working. Why is it so? Putting it down on paper allows you to take a closer look at patterns of behavior and areas you can focus on to improve the ones that you know are continuing to help you grow. You will also begin to see where you need to let go.

When in doubt about a relationship, run a few thoughts about it through the Thought Model. What are the feelings that come up? What are the actions you take as a result? It is so important when looking at how we show up, to really question our own motives for staying in relationships. If it's healthy and supportive, more times than not, the feelings it evokes should be positive.

Get a coach, or therapist, or counselor to help if you are feeling conflicted about the energy you have surrounding you. It is important to obtain an objective perspective especially if you feel too close to see the forest from the trees.

Chapter Ten

Find the Spark
Ignite your creativity.

When I stopped drinking I immediately felt something inside of me wake up. I'd been dulling the edges and keeping my feelings dormant for over two decades, so it was no surprise that once my mind began to clear, I suddenly had to pay attention to a lot of information coming to the surface. It's as if this information had been tucked away in my mind, waiting for the self-medicating to stop so I could let it out.

What came alive was my need to write. I had always been a big reader, but never had the urge to put pen to paper, so this sudden burst of energy that came over me was quite a surprise. I not only felt compelled to do it, I was literally obsessed with getting these words and ideas out into the world. I would wake up in the morning and my thoughts felt like they were on speed. At first, I seriously thought I was going nuts.

To calm these overwhelming feelings, I decided the best way to make sense of it was to start capturing it in a journal. That lasted about three days and when I faced the fact that I am simply not a journal writer, I pulled out my laptop and started typing. At first I used it as my own self-therapy, keeping it to myself. Then I realized that there was substance in my writing and it was centered around empowerment and inspiration—the two things I had been longing to access all my life. Coincidence, I think not!

I had no idea where the words were coming from, but it was as if a voice inside me that had the answers all along suddenly decided to reveal itself and all its wisdom. As my writing continued and I became more comfortable with it, I decided to let it serve a higher purpose than just my own healing.

I posted my first inspirational blog in 2011 and since then, I never looked back. While my writing was born out of a desire to express myself and make sense of the changes that were happening within me, this creative outlet has proven to mean so much more.

It's given me the opportunity to come out of my shell, help other women find inspiration in their daily lives, and opened me up to feeling more grateful for the things in my life that have brought me this far. I look back now and wonder what I would have done if I hadn't listened to what I had to say and channel it out into the world. Writing has literally changed my life and provided me with inner strength that I never knew I had.

I recently had a client in retirement who had loved to sing when she was younger. Her passion for music and performing went dormant during her drinking days, and it was not until many years into her sobriety that she re-engaged with her love for theatre. She now spends her time volunteering as a music director for the community college and is uplifted with the difference she is making in helping others realize their gifts.

I've met countless other women who have channeled their sober energy into creative pursuits of all kinds. Regardless of how it shows up, it's always a worthy pursuit. It's important to note that creativity doesn't necessarily have to be in the arts—it can come in all shapes and sizes. It's found in how you look at life and where you find inspiration. It's the recognition of what makes your heart sing that can make all the difference.

Backlog

I'm a huge proponent of accessing creativity under any circumstance, but in recovery, I believe it cracks us open and allows the deeper healing to happen. In the process, we gradually look for different ways to express ourselves. When you get rid of your means to escape, there is nothing left but your truth, and sooner or later, I can assure you, it will catch up with you.

I call this our creative backlog. All the thoughts, ideas, and feelings that had gone unexpressed and muted during addiction are looking for the right outlet to bring them out into the world.

Inspiration

When I started my blog, I was looking for a way to inspire myself and others. I have always been interested in reading stories about adversity that lifts people up to be better and bolder human beings. As I've learned over the years, inspiration can come from anywhere and some of the real gems can be found in the most unlikely places.

I look at my experience in recovery and know without a doubt that it has given me the gift to recognize the subtle beauty hidden in the ordinary. Every day. It's because I stop to take a look. I pay attention. I am more grateful for the incredible feeling I get when I wake up in the morning feeling good, or the time I spend simply listening to someone else.

These are the moments that inspire us to be better to ourselves and to others. So, when you are looking for something to light your wick and wiggle your creative juju, think about the treasures you are finding every day. They are full of color and texture and so much more. Ripe for the taking and ready to be made into something extraordinary.

The Paradox

One would think that many of our greatest artists who struggled with substance abuse did their best work while loaded on alcohol or drugs. I would challenge that in saying that although I agree that the likes of Kerouac and Hemingway were literary greats in their own right, can you imagine what kind of masterpieces they may have been able to create if they were firing on all cylinders? It is pretty mind blowing when you think about it.

Some may argue that alcohol offers up the liquid courage necessary to speak your mind, or let the words fall onto the page, or out into the world in whatever form you choose. But I believe true and authentic self-expression comes from an open heart and clear mind.

Creativity provides us with many things, but being able to express ourselves through any modality brings us to a place where the need to let it out trumps self-consciousness. Writing this book is a good example of how coupling the power of my own experience with creative expression can create something in service of others.

How do you best express yourself? Is it through writing or drawing, singing or dancing? Is it in listening to others and offering support? It may not be an obvious one. It could be through volunteering or in support of others' creative pursuits. Whatever it is, allowing yourself to let go and begin to explore what makes you tick is just the beginning. You will become more comfortable in listening to your inner muse, and before you know it, you will tap into something wonderful.

One of my favorite quotes by Elizabeth Gilbert is *"Create whatever causes a revolution in your heart., The rest of it will take care of itself."*

Words to live by.

The BS

I've never been very creative. I wouldn't know how to even get started. All of my creativity happened when I was younger. I don't have any burning desire to share anything. I'm afraid if I go there, too much of myself will be exposed.

Blockers

Don't be your own blocker. There are plenty of naysayers out there—don't be your own critic. I know, it's easier said than done, but self-doubt is always going to be there. Doing what lights you up, for your own joy and sense of satisfaction is all that matters.

The Shift

Coming into my own in recovery is about expression. In whatever form that takes for me, it is worth exploring. All it takes is an interest and the curiosity to explore it further. Creativity comes in so many forms and can be a private or public thing—it's up to me. The important part is letting it flow and releasing the creative energy that has been held back for so long.

Daily Practice

The first step in tapping into your creativity is to get comfortable with quiet and listen to yourself. I know, this may not always be easy, so bear with me on this one. The best way to access the energy that needs to surface is by being still and recognizing what your heart is telling you.

If you are able to meditate, it can bring forth the silence that helps draw up thoughts and feelings that will tell you something. It could be a thought, an idea, a word, a poem, or a prayer. Whatever it is, go with it.

The gut urges that you have are telling you something. Mine used to come in bursts of activity that typically followed moments where I was able to sit still and listen to my thoughts. It came through more clearly the more time

I spent grounding myself and being comfortable in those moments of self-reflection.

Keep a journal, join an interest group, paint, help a neighbor, take photographs. Whatever it is that is fun and effortless for you is the best place to start. No one even has to see the outcome. It's in the releasing that the healing and the brilliance happens.

Chapter Eleven

Bring It

Share all you've got. The world is waiting.

S t Ignatius Gymnasium, 1978

It was our sixth grade girls' basketball playoffs and we were playing St Ignatius. They were the team to beat. Strong and relentless, these girls knew how to play and came to win. They were serious and not there to fool around, and we knew every time we were up against them, we had to bring our A game.

Mr. Prenta was a coach with steadfast charisma. He seemed to appear mysteriously one day as if dropped on the steps of our school, ready to put our team on the map. He was a stocky guy with greased back hair and piercing brown eyes. He always had an unsmoked cigarette behind one ear and a mischievous grin that ran across his face after he'd tell a bad joke. Which unfortunately happened far too often. He was a retired athlete, unlikely to say the least, but he knew the game and there was an intensity about him that made you want to make him proud.

I was his starting guard for one reason only. I was quick and scrappy. I had absolutely no form whatsoever when I shot the ball, but I had speed. I could bob and weave and make it down the court in record time, so I got to play a lot.

This was an away game and we'd been down since the start. I was having an off day, had given up the ball a few times, and knew I wouldn't be in much longer. The clock was running down and getting closer to half time. At 12 points behind and 10 seconds left on the clock, Mr. Prenta called a time out. As we gathered in our huddle, I suddenly felt the sharpness of his gaze land on me as his hands firmly grabbed my shoulders and spun me around. He looked me square in the eye and said, "Ok, I want you to run the ball down to half court and then just give it all you got." I looked at him utterly confused and said, "You want me to do what?" He replied, "I want you to get to half court and just lob the ball toward the net with everything you've got. Don't even think about it, kid. Just lob it."

The swiftness of his delivery left me with no time to respond, let alone argue. I remember walking back toward the court feeling a mixture of slight amusement that quickly gave way to complete panic as I stepped inside the line.

I caught the ball as planned and started dribbling down court. I knew his plan had no teeth and it was a laughable long shot but he had picked me to send a message that regardless of the odds, we were in it for the long haul, so I had to do my best. I ran past half court and as I started to gain momentum, I hurled the ball into the air with all my might. The crowd let out a gasp as I felt it leave my hands and start swirling through the air. I remember feeling a twinge of relief at the distance it picked up hoping that my attempt wasn't a complete disaster and turned to start walking toward the bench. As I turned my gaze, I saw my teammates still looking down court and out of the corner of my eye, I caught a glimpse of the ball sink with a loud *whoosh* right through the net!

The sidelines cheered and my entire team let out a roar as they ran over to congratulate me. I was completely stunned. It was the first time I had ever felt such a remarkable sense of effortless strength. A rush of exhilaration and disbelief came over me and the first thought that popped into my head as we loaded into the van was, *I wish my parents had been here to see this*. As if having them witness it somehow would make it more real. They were proud nonetheless and although telling the story was nothing compared to the excitement on the court that day, I knew it was a moment I would never forget.

That's what happens when we decide to give it our all. Even in the most unlikely of circumstances we can at any given time, be called upon to let go of our fear and just let 'er rip. When we go all in, even if it feels like a futile or fruitless effort, taking action is all that matters.

By the way, if you're wondering if I ever went on to play professional basketball after that, I have to say, sadly no. In eighth grade, I moved on to gymnastics and after realizing I had absolutely no flexibility, I hung up my passion for exercise until well after my crazy days of college. Then in the early '90s I got into Jazzercise. Ok, totally dating myself and I promise my obsession was fleeting. But for any of you who may have dabbled in the craze, it was a great little workout!

The point is, whether it's in sports or any other pursuit, going for it takes more of a foundation than we sometimes think. To say just "get out there and make things happen" can feel daunting to those of us who may just be getting back into the game of life and reawakening to our own power. We need time to feel our own strength and come to terms with what we are here to do now, as sober individuals living in a world that can truly use what we have to offer.

The key to tapping into "all you've got" is figuring out what makes you come alive.

Meaning

Finding meaning in your life can feel overly complicated if you don't grasp the basic understanding that it is simply a choice you make. To apply meaning, you need to believe there is a plan for you and be open to the notion that whatever experiences you've had are leading you down a path to greater awareness.

The feeling of change and discomfort in early recovery can make this awareness more difficult to grasp. But the more you continue down your path, the more critical it becomes.

For those of us who consider ourselves empaths, or highly sensitive individuals, this connection may be easier to make. We feel energy more acutely and can sense a bigger picture more readily than most.

In fact, the initial reason some of us turned to alcohol in the first place is in an attempt to dull the inputs we encounter on a daily basis. Our senses are highly responsive not only to outside stimulus, but to the energy we absorb around us. When this is happening at a rapid pace, day in and day out, it can get overwhelming. Much like the sights and sounds of a Vegas casino, the input tends to overload our system.

On an intuitive level, we may know we're meant to play at a higher level out in the world, but on a practical level, it can be a bit more challenging to grasp this notion.

A critical mistake we make is deciding that our sobriety is a terrible curse that has been brought upon us. I can't tell you how many forums I have read and people I speak with who look at recovery as some curse or misfortune, or as an excuse to remain stuck in repetition of their story. I don't discount what they've gone through, I just think we need to start utilizing the lessons we learn from this pain in different ways if we are ever going to move beyond it.

Instead of listening to ourselves rehash our past challenges, why not put them to good use and start channeling our newfound energy to create an inspiring future.

Consider that as part of your healing process, you have been given a gift of grand proportions. You can take all of the heartache and pain of the past and transform it into your future in remarkable ways. Being in recovery allows you to take your experience and grow into the person we were meant to become.

Sobriety is the path that has been put in front of you and finding meaning in your calling is the best way to utilize it to its fullest.

Purpose

Thinking about purpose can be a whole new and seemingly unattainable concept once we enter recovery. Our relentless preoccupation with booze for so many years didn't leave us with much time for contemplation, let alone the desire to ponder what fires us up.

Once we come into the light of recovery for a period of time, our sense of self starts to peek through and we begin to start thinking about how we can contribute in the world as sober and participating adults.

The word "purpose" can sound so daunting. It's similar to the word "passion." There is a dramatic tone attached that makes us think of some profound event that needs to happen in order for it to come into view. As if the clouds will part and you'll suddenly know what it is. It doesn't happen quite like that, at least not for most people.

Purpose typically unfolds within the most unobvious of circumstances and gains momentum slowly and steadily as you continue to follow the path that brings you joy in your life.

Your purpose can be to help others, to fulfill your life's dream, or simply be one in the same. There is no real formula. It is merely an understanding of what you can contribute joyfully to the world. The good news is that life experience awakens our purpose, as long as we remain open to allow it to do so.

Connection

Finding connection in addiction often feels close to impossible and the farthest thing from our mind is to want to get back in the mix, but it is critical in recovery.

I still struggle with this. I am a highly sensitive introvert. Go figure. I am lucky enough to have a job that's all about connection, because left to my own devices I am afraid I would succumb to my reclusive tendencies.

It is not so easy for those of us who used to isolate in our drinking to seek out community when we first get sober because one of our favorite things to do was hide out. We'd prefer to fade into the background rather than get back out there and face the world.

One of the most difficult things for us to do when we are newly sober is to reach out to others. We feel raw and uncomfortable, and the last thing we want to do is start creating more drama in our lives by inviting more people in. We would much rather hang by ourselves and feel lonely than try to get out there and mix things up.

It is however, the first step in giving your light to others. When you share your truth, your heartaches, and triumphs, you are coming into your own and out of the darkness. It's an investment you are making in yourself in order to grow and evolve in recovery.

I encourage you to seek out a community that feels right for you. For recovery based groups, there are plenty of forums out there, but opportunities to connect with others in person on a regular basis is important. For those of you in AA, that may happen for you in the rooms. For others, it may be Women for Sobriety or SMART Recovery. For yoga enthusiasts, Recovery 2.0 and Y12SR are great options as well as She Recovers and of course my favorite, Sober Moxie that offer a variety of recovery resources and programs.

For general opportunities to find community, it's best to consider your interests and what type of collective you want to be a part of or would like to start yourself.

Sharing what you have with the world is risky. There's no doubt about it. It requires energy to give it all you've got and guts to face potential failure. But when we know we are here to serve others for a higher purpose, the reward far outweighs the potential downside.

It's as simple as that.

The BS

I have no idea what I want to do with my life. I don't have time to dream, I'm just concentrating on getting through my day. I don't have anything to give others. I could never change my career now. Things are stable and easy, there's no sense in rocking the boat.

Blockers

We are all tied down by jobs we may not love, or obligations we feel are keeping us from our true purpose. The world is going to continuously throw curve balls our way and the more we buy into the "shoulds" in life, the less likely we will be in finding purpose in what we do. We think we should be in a 9-5 job. We need to pay the bills. This typically drowns out our inner voice that may be screaming to us that we are meant to be working with kids or owning our own business. These perceived road blocks are merely self-imposed expectations we've been carrying around with us like saddle bags for too many years.

The Shift

I can't let my own inner judgment get the best of me. Sometimes purpose reveals itself after a series of events bring to light what I'm meant to do with greater clarity. There is no magic bullet, but the more I follow my heart, the more likely I am to find purpose and put a plan into action to start living in alignment with it.

Daily Practice

Jot down the activities that make you happy, the work you love, the causes that you feel passionate about, the people you like to surround yourself with, and your favorite pastimes. The more you know what you enjoy spending your time doing, the closer you get to determining where your true passion lies.

Chapter Twelve

Putting it All Together
The gems you've collected.

The truth of the matter is there's no more time to waste. You have to take advantage of the gifts that have been left at your doorstep. You have a tremendous opportunity to share your experience with the world in whatever way you see fit. It doesn't matter what it looks like. You just need to do it. Now, I'm not telling you to spill your story to every person you pass on the street, but the precious perspective you have gained from your life experiences is worth sharing and has primed you for a remarkable opportunity. To show up differently. To spread your wings and take flight, once and for all.

The gems you walk away with on the other side of addiction are countless, but I picked out some of my favorites to leave you with because I think they are some of the most valuable.

Clarity

You now have clarity. This is something you haven't had in a long time. The frame comes into focus and you realize what you've been missing. Colors seem brighter, textures are more interesting, your sense of smell and taste have changed. Most importantly, you're able to see yourself in the right light. You feel different and alive and full of greater dimension. You're ready to take this clarity and apply it to everything you do.

Nuance

You now have nuance. Drinking took away the grey area. It forced you to see in black and white, good or bad. For some of you, it made you steadfast in your resolve to block people out of your life who were not suiting your needs and you had a very difficult time forgiving.

Your perspective has shifted and life has become far less dramatic. Allowing you to think rationally and make decisions based on thoughtful introspection rather than raw reaction. You no longer see in extremes. You are more patient and willing to accept other's mistakes. You see all sides and in times like these, this unique perspective is more important than ever.

Honesty

You now have honesty. Freedom at its finest. This is one of my favorites because in recovery there is no other choice. You may have spent time in the past wrestling with a mess of lies and carrying around the shame of not being truthful to those you love. You're on a new path now. One that allows you to speak from the heart, regardless of the circumstances. Offering you a golden opportunity to unapologetically show people who you really are.

Connection

You now have connection. With yourself and with others. You no longer see this as an obstacle. You have the ability to connect and share and love those around you on a deeper level. You're able to understand the rumblings inside and have compassion with them as they surface. No longer afraid of their power and in a state of awareness you never thought possible. Emotion is your teacher and you are now an open and willing student.

Balance

You now have balance. What was once a constant state of unrest is now a place of awareness. In your mind and body, you have the ability to bring yourself into a space of calm at any time. No longer rocked by the unsteady energy of your past, you are grounded in your own knowing that life shows you what you're made of and time is your greatest healer.

Time

You now have time. It used to elude you. Untethered by addiction, time has taken on a whole new meaning. You understand the importance of remaining calm and present. It is expansive and giving. It allows you to do what you need to do in this world. It offers you the space to learn and grow. It's indeed on your side.

Freedom

You now have freedom. You are no longer tangled up in a self-created web of drama and anxiety. You have built a foundation that gives you the confidence to stand on your own and create a life that supports your recovery without distraction. You see this creation of angst as an unnecessary waste of precious energy. You choose what plays out between your ears and create your own outcomes.

Purpose

You now have purpose. In your past this didn't seem possible. All of your suffering and pain has brought you to a place of forgiveness and acceptance. It all happened for a reason. So that you could find your place in this world and expand what you have to give. It's now time for you to accept how precious your experience has been and use it to bring light to others.

As you well know, recovery is a strange and puzzling process, and it's certainly not a planned destination. Most of us enter into it in a state of complete and utter confusion. We've hit a point in our lives where continuing to self-destruct is no longer an option. We know sobriety is the solution but in the early stages, we are still trying to make sense of the problem that forced us there in the first place. It's not until we start healing that the good stuff begins to reveal itself.

Now that you're here. I say this with heaps of love, support and respect. It's time for you to recognize that you've survived for a reason. It is not because you're broken. It's quite the opposite. It's because you've been chosen. There is a reason you were put in this predicament. You were led astray in order to find your way back to a place of greater love and self-acceptance.

On a recent trip to India, I had a rare opportunity to meet with the wise and dedicated teacher, Sadhvi Bhagawati Saraswati at The Parmarth Niketan Ashram in Rishikesh who spoke about addiction. She said "In addiction, you were seeking the same spiritual destination as everyone else, you just got on the wrong train."

Your journey may have had its twists and turns, but as you can see, the destination still awaits you. You will never be at a loss for the blessings in your life. Your recovery has opened you up to an entirely new world filled with different expectations and opportunities. You have a richness inside you that has been honed over the years and you are strong and capable of manifesting anything you want in this life.

Now, it's entirely up to you to determine what that is and just how amazing it's going to be.

Godspeed, my friend.

THE *leap* TRUTHS

Surrender	It will set you free
Feel the Force	It's all around you.
Dig Deep	Honor your feelings. They're your best teachers.
Stay Present	It's just a matter of time.
Crush the Bubble	Keep thoughts that serve and lose the rest.
Sing Mama Sing	Let your voice be heard.
Breathe	Mindfulness is magic.
Take Care	You owe it to yourself and others.
Moxie Baby	Live on your own terms. Make it non-negotiable
Find the Spark	Awaken your creativity.
Bring It	Share all you've got. The world is waiting.

Acknowledgements

A special thanks to Alida Schuyler for spending her Sunday mornings teaching me what it means to be a powerful recovery coach.

Thanks to Tommy and Kia for their encouragement, wisdom and guidance at a time when I needed it most.

Thanks to Brooke Castillo who taught me that that I hold the power to change the outcomes in my life.

Thanks to my friends and family who have provided unwavering love and support throughout this process.

Finally, to the writers, coaches and teachers I have learned from over the years. Without whom this book would have never been written.

To the Morgan James Publishing team: Special thanks to David Hancock, CEO & Founder for believing in me and my message. To my Author Relations Manager, Margo Toulouse, thanks for making the process seamless and easy. Many more thanks to everyone else, but especially Jim Howard, Bethany Marshall, and Nickcole Watkins.

About the Author

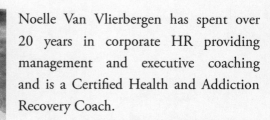

Noelle Van Vlierbergen has spent over 20 years in corporate HR providing management and executive coaching and is a Certified Health and Addiction Recovery Coach.

She is the founder of Sober Moxie, an addiction recovery coaching practice and in addition to her blog she is the creator of The Spark Salon, an inspirational resource that encourages women to ignite their lives.

She's made it her mission to help women recognize that this path is not just about sobriety, it's about embracing change and being bolder in all aspects of their lives. All it takes is support and the will to make it happen.

Noelle lives in San Jose, CA and loves adventure travel, reading, writing, photography, and hiking with her rambunctious pup Charlie.

Thank You

How close to your Truth are you?

Go to sobermoxie.com/book and complete the Leap Truths Assessment to identify your strengths and the areas that could be holding you back from living an amazing life in recovery.

Once you have a chance to review your results, let's connect to discuss ways to take your recovery to the next level.

One truth at a time.

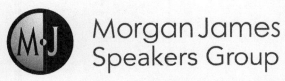

Morgan James
Speakers Group

www.TheMorganJamesSpeakersGroup.com

We connect Morgan James published authors with live and online events and audiences who will benefit from their expertise.

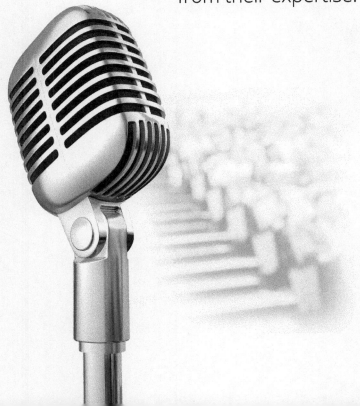

CPSIA information can be obtained
at www.ICGtesting.com
Printed in the USA
BVHW04s2324160518
516408BV00008B/708/P

9 781683 507376